MEDICAL INTELLIGENCE UNIT

TUMOR-INFILTRATING LYMPHOCYTES IN HUMAN MALIGNANCIES

Theresa L. Whiteside, Ph.D.

University of Pittsburgh School of Medicine
and the Pittsburgh Cancer Institute

R.G. LANDES COMPANY
AUSTIN

Medical Intelligence Unit

TUMOR-INFILTRATING LYMPHOCYTES IN HUMAN MALIGNANCIES

R.G. LANDES COMPANY
Austin

CRC Press is the exclusive worldwide distributor of publications of the Medical Intelligence Unit.
CRC Press, 2000 Corporate Blvd., NW, Boca Raton, FL 33431. Phone: 407/994-0555.

Submitted: July 1993
Published: September 1993

Production Manager: Carol Harwell
Copy Editor: Constance Kerkaporta

Printed on recycled paper by Armstrong Printing Co., Austin, Texas, U.S.A.

Please address all inquiries to the Publisher:
R.G. Landes Company, 909 Pine Street, Georgetown, TX 78626
or
P.O. Box 4858, Austin, TX 78765
Phone: 512/ 863 7762; FAX: 512/ 863 0081

ISBN 1-879702-78-9
CATALOG # LN0278

Library of Congress Cataloging-in-Publication Data

Whiteside, Theresa L., 1939-
Tumor-infiltrating lymphocytes in human malignancies / Theresa L. Whiteside.
p. cm.—(Medical intelligence unit)
Includes bibliographical references and index.
ISBN 1-879702-78-9 (hard cover) : $89.95
1. Tumors—Immunological aspects. 2. Lymphocytes. 3. Cancer cells—Growth. 4. Metastasis. I. Title. II. Series.
[DNLM: 1. Lymphocytes, Tumor-infiltrating. 2. Neoplasms—immunology. QZ 200 W588 1993]
QR188.6.W48 1993
616.99'2079—dc20
DNLM/DLC 93-20908
For Library of Congress CIP

CONTENTS

1. Introduction 1

2. In Situ Characterization of TIL 6

3. Methods for Isolation of TIL from Human Solid Tumors 32

4. Morphologic and Phenotypic Characteristics of Freshly Isolated TIL 39

5. Functional Characteristics of Fresh TIL 52

6. In Vitro Expansion and Characteristics of Cultured TIL 67

7. TIL and Their Role in Tumor Surveillance and Progression 81

8. Adoptive Immunotherapy with TIL 89

Index 111

FOREWORD AND ACKNOWLEDGMENT

This book is about tumor-infiltrating lymphocytes. An explanation might be in order to account for my long-standing preoccupation with the cells that accumulate at the site of tumor growth or metastasis. As a clinical immunologist I have long believed that studies performed with human peripheral blood lymphocytes (PBL), representing but a small fraction of lymphocytes responsible for host defense and immune competence, are inadequate or even misleading. Immune events most relevant to the pathophysiology of disease occur not in the blood but in tissues. However, tissue-infiltrating lymphocytes are not readily accessible in humans, and available biopsy material generally yields only a small number of cells for evaluation. On the other hand, it appeared to me that tumors are an ideal source of tissue-infiltrating lymphocytes, and in order to pursue this idea I went on sabbatical to Ludwig Institute for Cancer Research in Lausanne, Switzerland. In 1984 and 1985 Lorenzo Moretta and his group were there cloning and functionally characterizing human T lymphocytes, and Jean-Charles Cerottini, Director of the Institute, had a strong immunology program in place. So, with invaluable assistance from Sylvia Miescher, a postdoctoral fellow at Ludwig at that time, and Vladimir von Fliedner, in whose laboratory I was situated, we began a series of studies with human TIL that led to an improved understanding of TIL function and their immunobiology. I have continued these studies at the Pittsburgh Cancer Institute with encouragement from Ronald Herberman and in collaboration with various postdoctoral fellows who have succeeded one another in my laboratory over the years. In the course of our studies TIL have become prominent, and the issue of their use or usefulness in cancer therapy has generated a flurry of excitement and controversy that continues unabated today. Steven Rosenberg and his group at the Surgery Branch of NCI deserve credit for championing TIL as therapeutically important cells and promoting their application to immunotherapy of cancer. In a small way we have contributed to the overall effort of trying to define the role of TIL in tumor growth and metastasis. In this book I hope to convey to the reader some of the feelings of excitement, scientific curiosity, satisfaction and disappointment that have accompanied me during the TIL quest. To see TIL in clinical trials and to witness and participate in the development of this form of therapy has been a tremendously exciting and rewarding experience. My expectation is that TIL will remain an object of intensive investigation in the future to further establish their clinical efficacy and optimize TIL therapy. I would like to thank my husband, Thomas M. Howe Nimick, Jr., for his continuing interest and support and for living with TILs, as it were, for many years. My postdoctoral fellows, Drs. D.S. Heo, S. Takagi, Y.L. Wang, Y. Shimizu, L. Vaccarello, E. Weidmann, D. Vitolo, S. Yasumura, H. Hirabayashi, W.-C. Lin and E. Letessier, have all significantly contributed to the work I describe, and I thank them for all their efforts. My secretary, Cheryl Michel, has been instrumental in completing this book, and her commitment and help are gratefully acknowledged. Also, I am grateful to my staff and colleagues at the Pittsburgh Cancer Institute, Drs. E. Elder, N. Vujanovic, H. Rabinowich, Mrs. D. Friberg and Miss Jeanne Nepa, all of whom have contributed in various meaningful ways to this project. Many experiments described in this book were performed at my laboratory, the Immunologic Monitoring and Diagnostic Laboratory of the Pittsburgh Cancer Institute. I wish to thank the staff of the laboratory for their help and dedication. Finally, I want to thank the National Office of the American Cancer Society for providing two generous grants in support of our TIL work (IM-588 and IM-696).

Theresa L. Whiteside, Ph.D.

CHAPTER 1

INTRODUCTION

Infiltrations of mononuclear cells (MNC), which are commonly seen at or around the site of tumor growth or metastasis, are mainly composed of lymphocytes and macrophages.[1-3] This type of chronic inflammatory infiltrate may be replaced in some tumors or in certain areas of tumors by granulocytic acute infiltrate.[4] The proportion of lymphocytes to macrophages in MNC infiltrates present in tissues immediately surrounding the tumors or in the tumor stroma is variable from one tumor type to another.[5,6] The lymphocytic component of the infiltrate consists mostly of T cells, and B lymphocytes are only rarely a significant component of the infiltrate.[1,6] In some carcinomas, plasma cells may be present and represent a substantial infiltrating element.[7] Pathologists have long been aware of the presence of MNC infiltrates in the tumor stroma, and, over the years, the role of these infiltrates in tumor growth or metastasis and their influence on patient prognosis or survival have been a subject of considerable controversy. Histology has indeed been useful in providing clues regarding cellular identity, localization and intensity of these infiltrates. It was on the basis of histologic observations that MacCarty first suggested in 1922 that lymphoid infiltration in breast tumors was a sign of host resistance.[8] In the mid-1970s, Underwood[9] and then Ioachim[10] proposed that MNC infiltrates in human tumors may have a direct relationship to improved prognosis and may represent an expression of immune surveillance. According to the proposal, large infiltrations with MNC into a solid tumor might be indicative of the vigorous local inflammatory response, with an accompanying accumulation of immune effector cells, some of which might represent an autotumor (AuTu)-specific component of the infiltrate.

Over the years, the idea that tumor-infiltrating lymphocytes (TIL) are not just inflammatory cells but rather are effector cells, which might be specifically recruited to the tumor as a part of antitumor immune surveillance mechanism, has been attractive to immunologists and has led to a vigorous search for the presence of AuTu-specific cytotoxic T lymphocytes (CTL) among TIL. Intuitively, whether TIL are considered to be nonspecific inflammatory cells or AuTu-specific effector cells, their presence in the tumor should be associated with a better prognosis in comparison to tumors devoid of TIL, based on the ability of either of these cell populations to mediate antitumor effects. However, although several studies such as those by Svennevig et al,[11] Watt and House,[12] and others[13-16] emphasized better survival for patients whose tumors were well infiltrated with MNC, many other studies were unable to find any positive correlation between the intensity of lymphoid infiltrates and prognosis for better survival. This lack of a clear-cut correlation created a need for a reasonable explanation as to why MNC accumulated in the tumor and to what extent their functional characteristics reflected the presence of antitumor effector cells. In view of this lack of significant and consistent association between the intensity of MNC infiltrates and prognosis for survival in most situations, a consideration was given to the possibility that in addition to intensity, a composition as well as activation and functional properties of the infiltrating cells might contribute to their impact on tumor growth or metastasis. Infiltrating MNC are known to be a source of multiple cytokines, many of which have growth potentiating properties for tissue and perhaps tumor cells.[17] It is now also known that tumor cells express receptors for a variety of cytokines,[18-20] and the possibility has to be considered that infiltrating MNC could promote tumor growth. In fact, this possibility has been discussed in the literature long before cytokines have been discovered.[21] Furthermore, human solid tumors may be a source of immunosuppressive factors, which would tend to suppress antitumor functions of infiltrating MNC. Therefore, multiple interactions between the tumor and infiltrating cells might determine the outcome of the malignant or metastatic process. It is possible that the controversy about the prognostic significance of MNC in the tumor can be at least partially explained by the complexity of interactions existing between the various cell types in the tumor microenvironment and by the ability of the infiltrating cells to produce tumor growth-promoting as well as tumor growth-inhibiting cytokines.

With the advent of immunohistology in the 1980s, it was possible to ascertain that most tumor-infiltrating MNC had a T-cell phenotype.[22,23] The realization that T cells were the predominant component of TIL has focused attention on a possibility that T cells sensitized to tumor-associated antigens (TAA) selectively accumulate in human tumors. Results obtained in murine tumor models, where the presence of tumor-specific CTL, has been confirmed in several studies,[24,25] strongly supported this notion. To test the possibility that TIL in human solid tumors contained tumor-specific CTL, a number of studies has been initiated based on the ability to outgrow TIL in the presence of interleukin-2 (IL-2) either in bulk cultures or as clones derived from single cells and to test AuTu specificity of these cultured TIL. This approach was difficult to implement with TIL from human solid tumors, not only because of limited numbers of TIL that could be recovered from tumor biopsies, but primarily because of a requirement for fresh, viable autologous and allogeneic cell targets for in vitro sensitization (IVS) and to confirm cell specificity. The results of these studies indicated that TIL, isolated from human solid tumors and cultured with IL-2, were heterogeneous populations of mostly major histocompatibility complex (MHC)-unrestricted effector cells, but that AuTu-specific CTL might be present among TIL. These AuTu-specific CTL are difficult to outgrow from most human TIL, with a notable exception of TIL obtained from melanomas, where considerable evidence has accumulated for spontaneous outgrowth of CTL during long-term cultures with IL-2.[26,27]

In 1986, Rosenberg and his collaborators reported that TIL derived from a murine tumor and grown in the presence of IL-2 were 50-100 times more effective than lymphokine-activated killer (LAK) cells obtained from the spleen in eradicating established pulmonary or liver metastasis in a murine sarcoma model.[28] This finding led Rosenberg and his collaborators to initiate clinical trials with human TIL in order to evaluate clinical efficacy of adoptive immunotherapy (AIT) with TIL and IL-2 in patients with metastatic melanoma or renal cell carcinoma (RCC).[29,30] These clinical trials have generated enormous interest in TIL as a source of therapeutically superior cells. However, the initial optimism about TIL as a source of therapeutically useful cells had to be tempered by rather modest results of these clinical trials, in which over 70% of patients remained unresponsive to therapy.[29,30] Today, a healthy skepticism has developed in respect to the therapeutic effectiveness of human TIL. Advantages of AIT with TIL, as opposed to LAK cells or other cell populations of effector cells derived from the peripheral blood, are not quite clear in man. For example, it remains questionable whether TIL are indeed tumor-specific effector cells and whether TIL localize to the tumor site or to the tumor metastases following AIT. Above all, a relatively low frequency of responses, which have not been unequivocally higher than those obtained with cytokines alone, other adoptively transferred cells or with more conventional therapies, and an even smaller proportion of long-lasting responses following TIL therapy, have resulted in some disappointment and indicated a need for re-evaluation of TIL-based therapies. For these reasons, considerable efforts are now being made to provide both a strong rational basis for AIT with TIL and to improve its therapeutic efficacy. In spite of these setbacks, AIT with TIL remains one of the best characterized and, in some patients, clearly effective clinical approaches to immunotherapy of advanced metastatic cancer, particularly in patients who have failed previous conventional therapy.

Efforts to improve therapeutic efficiency of TIL have been mainly focused on genetic modification of the effector cells. Transfer of cytokine genes into TIL as well as therapy with TIL genetically-marked with, e.g., neomycin resistance (NeoR) gene, are being used to, respectively, improve effectiveness of the therapy and to test the ability of TIL to localize to the tumor site. These two goals are closely related because the principle of genetic alteration of TIL by transfection with cytokine genes is directly linked to the expectation that systemically-injected TIL will localize to the tumor site, thus, serving as a vehicle for delivery of cytokines to the tumor. However, evidence for selective accumulation of adoptively-transferred TIL at the tumor site is not as strong as to satisfy current criticism. The definitive experiment, in which localization to the tumor of TIL and autologous PBL, each population labeled with a distinct genetic marker, could be compared, has not yet been performed. It is necessary to recognize, nevertheless, that the ongoing attempts at evaluating therapeutic efficacy of TIL and defining the mechanism of the antitumor effects are necessary steps in validation and optimization of this form of therapy.

Although TIL from experimental murine tumors have been extensively studied and much has been learned from these studies, the purpose of this book is to provide an overview of TIL in human tumors. My objective is to assess not only phenotypic and functional properties of these cells, but to evaluate their biologic role in tumor growth and progression. In addition, the role of TIL in anticancer therapy following their in vitro expansion and activation in the presence of cytokines will be considered, as will more novel attempts at improving therapeutic efficacy of TIL. Considerable attention that TIL have received in recent years seems to be justified. Yet, a number of unanswered questions about TIL remain, and these are listed in Table 1. In view of a great deal of ambiguity and conflicting evidence with respect to the biologic role TIL may play in tumor growth and metastasis, it seems reasonable to try and resolve the conflict through scientific investigation. On the other hand, the initial promise offered by AIT with TIL, which has emerged as a novel and promising

Table 1. Unanswered questions about tumor-infiltrating lymphocytes[a]

1. What is the role of TIL in control of tumor growth or metastasis?
2. Are TIL enriched in AuTu-specific CTL relative to PBL?
3. Can therapeutically-useful TIL be "generated" from all types of human tumors?
4. Do adoptively-transferred TIL preferentially localize to the tumor?
5. How to ex vivo tailor TIL for optimal antitumor effects?

[a] Abbreviations: TIL = tumor-infiltrating lymphocytes; CTL = cytolytic T lymphocytes; PBL = peripheral blood lymphocytes; AuTu = autologous tumor.

approach to treatment of at least some patients with metastatic disease unresponsive to conventional therapies,[29,30] has focused attention of the clinician on TIL. Today, this therapeutic modality remains highly visible. The potential and limitations of TIL therapy and the future of this form of therapy will be critically assessed based on currently available evidence from the recently completed clinical trials with TIL as well as newer information about the immunobiology of these cells. It is hoped that through a better understanding of TIL as antitumor effector cells and of their role in the control of malignancy, the reader will obtain a comprehensive view of why these cells remain an attractive source of AuTu-specific effector cells and why so much effort is being expended to provide a rational experimental basis for their therapeutic use.

References

1. Vose BM, Moore M. Human tumor-infiltrating lymphocytes: A marker of host response. Semin Hematol 1985; 22:27-40.
2. Allen CA, Hogg N. Association of colorectal tumor epithelium expressing HLA-D/DR with CD8-positive T-cells and mononuclear phagocytes. Cancer Res 1987; 47:2919-2923.
3. Mantovani A. Tumor-associated macrophages. Current Opinion in Immunol 1990; 2:689-692.
4. Pretlow TP, Keith EF, Cryar AK, Bartolucci AA, Pitts AM, Pretlow TG, Kimball PM, Bookmaker EA. Eosinophil infiltration of human colon carcinoma as a prognostic indicator. Cancer Res 1987; 43:2997-3000.
5. Whiteside TL. Human tumor-infiltrating lymphocytes and their characterization. In: Lotzova E, Herberman RB., eds. Role of Interleukin 2 Activated Killer Cells in Cancer. Boca Raton: CRC Press, Inc., 1990: 133-151.
6. Whiteside TL, Jost LM, Herberman RB. Tumor-infiltrating lymphocytes: Potential and limitations to their use for cancer therapy. Crit Rev Oncol/Hematol 1992; 25-47.
7. Barnes L. Pathology of the head and neck: General considerations. In: Myers EN, Sueu JY., eds. Cancer of the Head and Neck. New York: Churchill Livingstone, 1989: 75-99.
8. MacCarty WC. Factors which influence longevity in cancer. Am Surg 1922; 76:9-12.
9. Underwood JCE. Lymphoreticular infiltration in human tumors: Prognostic and biological implications. A review. Br J Cancer 1974; 30:538-548.
10. Ioachim HL. The stroma reaction of tumors: An expression of immune surveillance. JNCI 1979; 57:465-475.
11. Svennevig JL, Lunde OC, Holter J, Bjorgsvik D. Lymphoid infiltration and prognosis in colorectal carcinoma. Br J Cancer 1984; 49:375-377.
12. Watt AG, House AK. Colonic carcinoma: A quantitative assessment of lymphocyte infiltration at the periphery of colonic tumors related to prognosis. Cancer 1978; 41:279-282.
13. Lauder I, Aherne W. The significance of lymphocytic infiltration in neuroblastoma. Br J Cancer 1972; 26:321-330.
14. Kreider JW, Bartlett GL, Butkiewicz BL. Relationship of tumor leucocytic infiltration to host defense mechanisms and prognosis. Cancer Met Rev 1984; 3:53-74.
15. Haskill S. Some historical perspectives on the relationship between survival and mononuclear cell infiltration. In: Haskill S., ed. Tumor Immunity and Prognosis: The Role of Mononuclear Cell Infiltration. New York: Marcel Dekker, 1982: 1-10.
16. Wolf G, Hudson J, Peterson K, Miller H, McClatchey KD. Lymphocyte subpopulations infiltrating squamous carcinomas of the head and neck: Correlations with extent of tumor and prognosis. Otolaryngol Head Neck Surg 1986; 95:142-152.
17. Schirrmacher V. Shifts in tumor cell phenotypes induced by signals from the microenvironment. Relevance for the immunobiology of cancer metastasis. Immunobiol 1980; 157:89-98.
18. Weidmann E, Sacchi M, Plaisance S, Heo DS, Yasumura S, Lin WC, Johnson JT, Herberman RB, Azzarone B, Whiteside TL. Receptors for interleukin 2 on human squamous cell carcinoma cell lines and tumor in situ. Cancer Res 1992; 52:5963-5970.
19. Baldwin GC, Gasson JC, Kaufman SE, Quan SG, Williams RE, Avalos BR, Gazdar AF, Golde DW, DiPersio JF. Nonhematopoietic

tumor cells express functional GM-CSF receptors. Blood 1989; 73:1033-1037.
20. Rimoldi D, Salvi S, Hartmann F, Schreyer M, Blum S, Zografos L, Plaisance S, Azzarone B, Carrel S. Expression of IL-2 receptors in human melanoma cells. AntiCancer Res 1993; 13:555-564.
21. Prehn RT, Main JM. Immunity to methylcholanthrene-induced sarcomas. JNCI 1957; 18:769-778.
22. Poppema S, Brocker EB, de Leij L, Terbrack D, Visscher T, Ter Haar A, Macher E, The TH, Sorg C. In situ analysis of the mononuclear cell infiltrate in primary malignant melanoma of the skin. Clin Exp Immunol 1983; 51:77-82.
23. Rowe DJ, Beverley PC. Characterization of breast cancer infiltrates using monoclonal antibodies to human leukocyte antigens. Br J Cancer 1984;49:149-159.
24. Brunner KT, MacDonald HR, Cerottini JC. Quantitation and clonal isolation of cytotoxic T lymphocyte precursors selectively infiltrating murine sarcoma virus-induced tumors. J Exp Med 1981;154:362-373.
25. Binz H, Fenner M, Engel R, Wigzell H. Studies on chemically induced rat tumors. II. Partial protection against syngeneic lethal tumors by cloned syngeneic cytotoxic T lymphocytes. Int J Cancer 1983;32:491-500.
26. Itoh K, Tilden AB, Balch CM. Interleukin 2 activation of cytotoxic T lymphocytes infiltrating into human metastatic melanomas. Cancer Res 1986;46:3011-3017.
27. Muul LM, Spiess PJ, Director EP, Rosenberg SA. Identification of specific cytolytic immune responses against autologous tumor in humans bearing malignant melanoma. J Immunol 1987;138:989-995.
28. Rosenberg SA, Spiess P, Lafreniere R. A new approach to adoptive immunotherapy of cancer with tumor-infiltrating lymphocytes. Science 1986;233:1318-1321.
29. Topalian SL, Solomon D, Avis FP, Chang AE, Freerksen DL, Linehan WM, Lotze MT, Robertson CN, Seipp CA, Simon P, Simpson CG, Rosenberg SA. Immunotherapy of patients with advanced cancer using tumor-infiltrating lymphocytes and recombinant interleukin-2: A pilot study. J Clin Oncol 1988;6:839-853.
30. Rosenberg SA, Packard BS, Aebersold PM, Solomon D, Topalian SL, Toy ST, Simon P, Lotze MT, Yang JC, Seipp CA, Simpson C, Carter C, Bock S, Schwartzentruber D, Wei JP, White DE. Use of tumor-infiltrating lymphocytes and interleukin-2 in the immunotherapy of patients with metastatic melanoma. A preliminary report. N Engl J Med 1988;319:1676-1680.

CHAPTER 2

In Situ Characterization of TIL

Information about the nature of cellular infiltrates present in the tumor can be obtained from microscopic observation of tumor tissues removed during surgery. In general, biopsy tissue is submitted to surgical pathology, fixed, embedded in paraffin, sectioned and examined by a pathologist for diagnosis. This type of routine histopathologic examination generally includes an overall estimation of the type and extent of inflammatory cells present but does not provide more specific details regarding the number, distribution or exact cellular composition of the infiltrates. To obtain such information, investigators are obliged to make a special effort. Often, the ability to correlate characteristics of the infiltrate with the tumor type, stage or pathologic grade is dependent on studies performed by the pathologist as a part of a research program. To characterize the phenotype of MNC in the tumor, biopsy tissue in excess of what is needed for diagnosis has to be available for frozen sections and immunohistologic techniques employed. While these techniques are now commonly available in most surgical pathology laboratories, only a few years ago they were considered to be in the research domain. As a consequence, data that are available regarding in situ characterization of TIL in various human tumors are not always reliable. Such data have come from individual series of studies performed over the last 30 or so years by various investigators from different geographic locations who employed somewhat different methodologies, frequently without much attention to quality controls. Not surprisingly, the findings were often dramatically different and, as described below, conclusions regarding the nature of infiltrates and their relationship to prognosis or survival of patients with cancer were often controversial.

In this chapter, a short summary of methodologies currently available for in situ characterization of TIL will be provided, followed by more complete evaluation of various methods and examples of their usefulness. The goal is to provide the reader not so much with a comprehensive review of research in this area but rather with an overview of the most important findings that have emerged from this research and with a commentary regarding in situ characterization of human TIL.

METHODS FOR IN SITU STUDIES OF TIL

There are three basic techniques available for in situ characterization of human TIL: histopathology, immunohistology, and in situ hybridization

(ISH). Of the three, *histopathology* is the oldest and the most widely used. Much of what is known about TIL localization, distribution, and density in human tumors has been derived from the examination of biopsy sections stained with conventional histologic reagents.[1,2] Although the histopathologist is generally more concerned with the presence and/or differentiation stage of the tumor cell in a biopsy specimen, histopathologic examination can yield important data about the inflammatory infiltrate. The chronic vs. acute nature of the infiltrate as well as the distribution of its lymphocytic vs. granulocytic components can be determined on conventional paraffin-embedded sections stained with hematoxylin and eosin (H&E). Furthermore, serial paraffin-embedded sections offer an opportunity to examine the distribution of inflammatory infiltrates in various areas of the same tumor. In examining histopathologic specimens for the degree and distribution of infiltrates in the tumor, the pathologist generally utilizes a scale designed to reflect different degrees of infiltration, based on the number of inflammatory cells/high power field (HPF). For example, a designation of 1+ can be applied to specimens containing less than 25% of inflammatory cells/HPF, while 4+ designates the presence of more than 75% of cells/HPF (see Fig. 1). This type of evaluation is highly subjective, of course, since it depends on individual pathologist's interpretation of the degree of infiltration in the specimen at hand. To avoid bias, more than two independent observers should perform the counts independently and report the combined counts. Whenever possible, morphometry should be substituted for visual examination of the slides, and morphometrically-determined numbers of inflammatory cells and their distribution in the specimen should be obtained. Morphometric measurements assure a fair degree of objectivity as well as a much greater precision in counting the infiltrating cells.

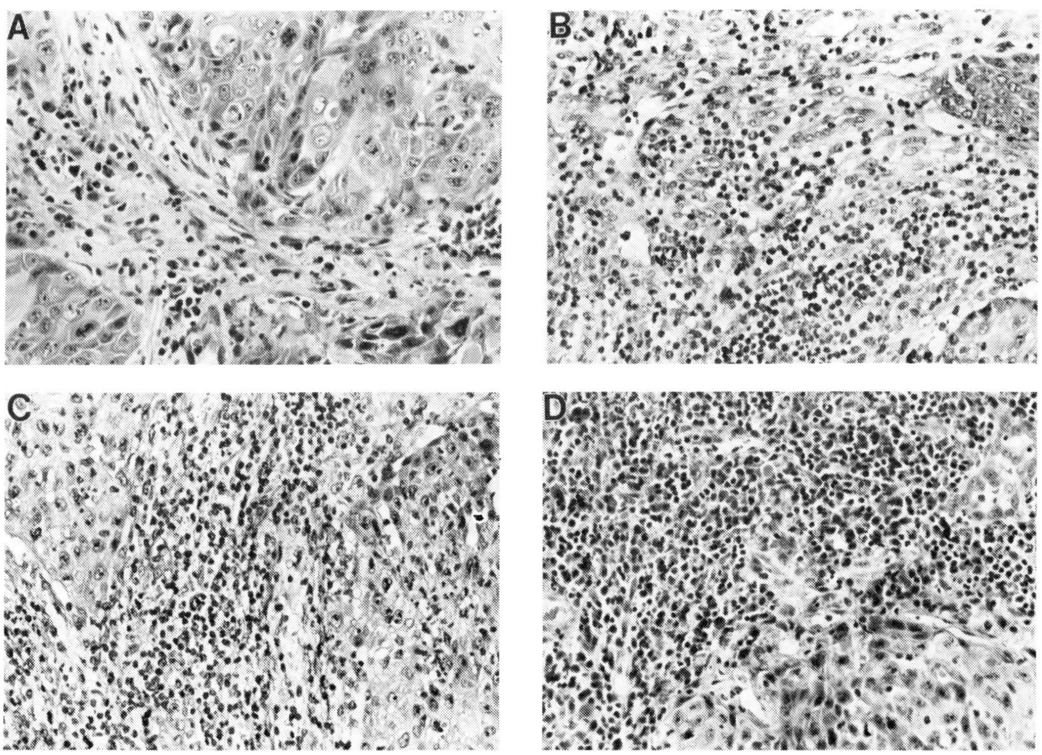

Fig. 1. Histopathology of squamous cell carcinoma of the head and neck. Intensity of mononuclear cell infiltrates into the stroma of four different tumors was graded as 1+ in a*; 2+ in* b*; 3+ in* c*; and 4 in* d*. Hematoxylin & eosin. Mag x 350.*

Immunohistology, utilizing labeled monoclonal antibodies (mAbs), specific for individual surface antigens (Ags) on infiltrating cells, was introduced in the late 1970s and has greatly facilitated the ability to define the phenotype of TIL. This methodology depends on the availability of well-characterized mAbs, each specific for a surface Ag expressed on human MNC. Today, such mAbs are readily available commercially from a variety of sources. Several serial cryostat sections, each stained with a different and carefully pretitered mAb, are employed for studies of TIL phenotype or localization. Immunohistology can be performed on sections of fixed and paraffin-embedded tissues, but only those surface Ags which survive fixation in formaldehyde and paraffin-embedding will give satisfactory results. Since many surface Ags on MNC do not survive such processing, cryosections are generally more reliable for immunohistology of TIL in situ. Immunostaining which, in the past, was mainly performed with fluorescein- or

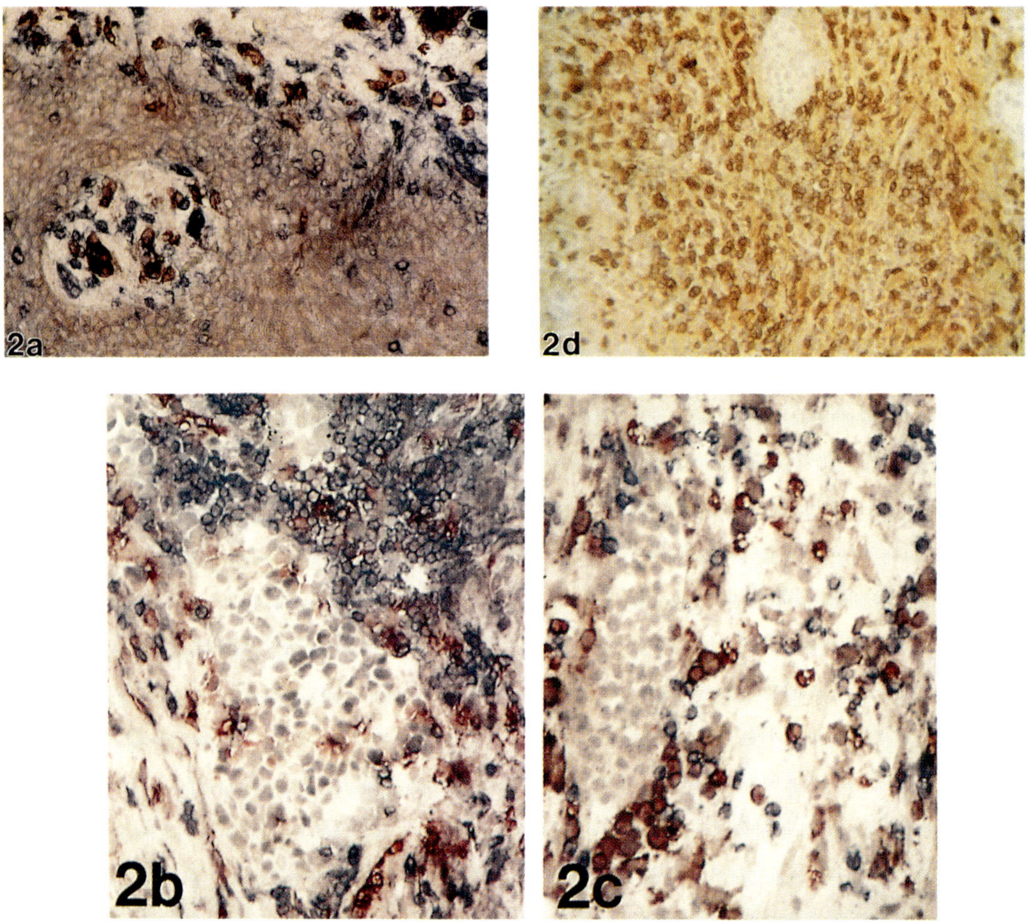

Fig. 2. Immunohistology of tumor-infiltrating lymphocytes (TIL) in cryostat tissue sections. In a, *TIL in a squamous cell carcinoma of the head and neck stained with anti-CD2 (blue) and anti-CD15 (red) mAbs by a double immunoenzymatic method. Note that both T cells (CD2⁺) and macrophages (CD15⁺) are infiltrating the tumor stroma and parenchyma. Mag x 750. In* b *and* c, *two sections of a malignant melanoma obtained from different areas of the tumor were stained as described above. Note that intense MNC infiltrate of predominantly blue (CD2⁺) cells is present around the nest of tumor cells in* b *and that in another area of the same tumor (c), the infiltrate is less intense and consists largely of red (CD15⁺) cells. Mag x 350 in* b; *x 400 in* c. *In* d, *a cryostat section of a breast carcinoma showing an intense infiltrate of CD3⁺ T lymphocytes in the tumor stroma. Mag x 350. Figures* b *and* c *were reproduced with permission from Chen et al, Lab Invest 1987;56:114-119.*

rhodamine-labeled mAbs, has recently been made highly sensitive by the use of sandwich techniques, employing antibodies labeled with enzymes or the avidin-biotin amplification system.[3] In addition, as shown in Figures 2 and 3, sequential applications of two mAbs, each labeled with a different enzyme now allow for the simultaneous visualization in tissue of cells expressing two different Ags.[4] Interpretation of immunostaining is again subjective, as it depends on microscopic examination by an observer who is expected to distinguish positive cells from background. Nonspecific staining may be a serious problem in some tissues, and the use of appropriate controls is obligatory in this methodology. The determination of the number of positive cells present in tissue is also difficult and time-consuming, as it depends on visual counts per each microscopic field examined, and its accuracy and objectivity is determined by the rigorousness of the investigator. Microscopic counts of cells in serial sections of the specimen, each section having been stained with a mAb specific for a different surface Ag, are likely to be biased, most often by a tendency of the investigator to select a field with a "right" number of conveniently distributed positive cells rather than a representative field. To avoid bias, immunoenzymatically-stained serial sections should be evaluated by video-image analysis.

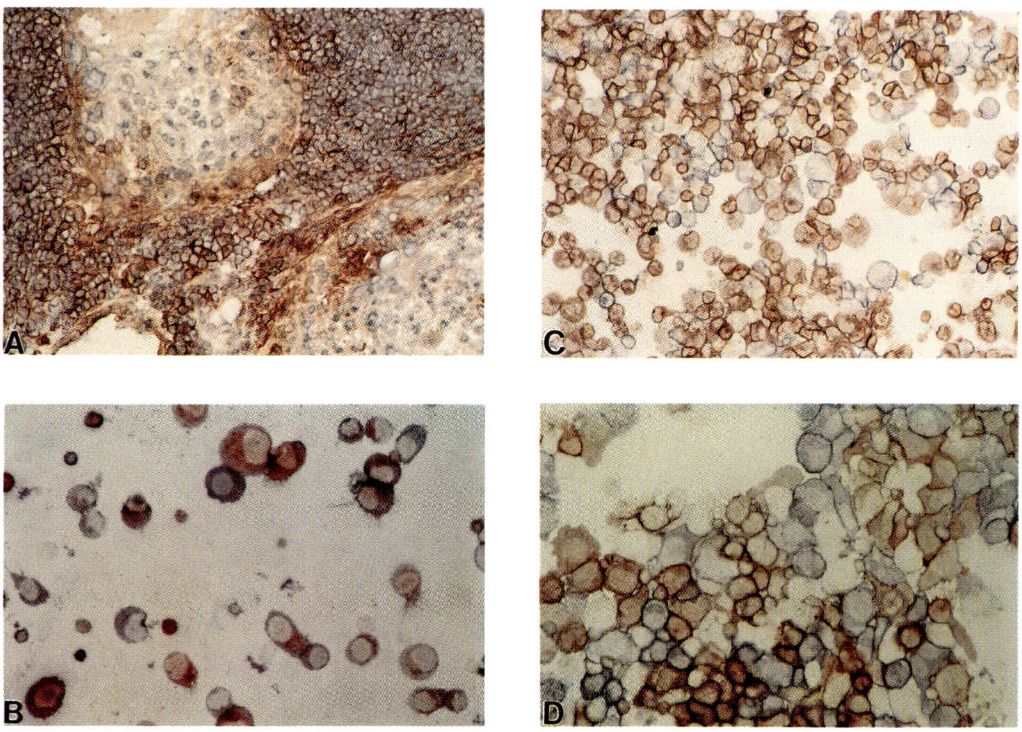

Fig. 3. Two-color immunohistology of tumor-infiltrating lymphocytes (TIL) in cryostat tissue sections. In a, TIL infiltrate in a squamous cell carcinoma of the head and neck (SCCHN) was stained with anti-CD3 (blue) and anti-HLA-DR (red) mAbs. Note an intense MNC infiltrate in the tumor stroma consisting of $CD3^+$ T lymphocytes many of which are also HLA-DR^+ (i.e., activated). Mag x 500. In b, TIL freshly obtained from a SCCHN were cytocentrifuged and stained with anti-CD3 and anti-HLA-DR mAbs. Note that many T cells (blue) are doubly stained with red, i.e., express HLA-DR. Mag x 1500. In c, TIL obtained from a patient with malignant melanoma were cultured for 3 weeks in the presence of IL-2, cytocentrifuged and stained with anti-CD8 (red) and anti-CD4 (blue) mAbs. Note that in this culture, $CD8^+$ lymphocytes predominated. Mag x 900. In d, TIL from another 3-week culture established with TIL obtained from a different patient with malignant melanoma. TIL were cytocentrifuged and stained as described above. Note that in this culture, $CD4^+$ (red) lymphocytes outnumber $CD8^+$ (blue) lymphocytes. Mag x 1200.

In examining TIL in situ by immunoenzymatic staining, it is important to bear in mind that the phenotype of a cell (e.g., $CD4^+$ vs. $CD8^+$ or $CD3^+CD25^+$ vs. $CD56^+$ DR^+) observed in situ does not provide information about its functional capacity. While immunologists are well attuned to this rule, pathologists may tend to interpret phenotypic characteristics in terms of functional attributes of a given lymphocyte. Such interpretation may, of course, be incorrect, and it is well to remember that the phenotype of TIL in situ must not be equated with their function. For example, while a proportion of TIL in situ express activation markers (CD25, HLA-DR; see Fig. 2), TIL are functionally immunosuppressed when first isolated from the tumor (see Chapter 5). Many investigators consider TIL in situ to be activated lymphocytes. Yet, expression of activation markers on TIL does not mean that these cells function as activated lymphocytes. Interpretation of immunohistologic data should always be made carefully and objectively with the goal of identifying differences in the phenotype, number, and distribution of TIL within each tumor examined.

The third technique that has only begun to be utilized recently for analysis of tumor-infiltrating MNC is *in situ hybridization* (ISH) with labeled cDNA probes, oligonucleotides or anti-sense RNA probes. This technology offers an opportunity to determine the expression of genes in TIL and in the tumor cells. Of special interest is the ability to measure the expression of cytokine genes in TIL or tumor cells, because it offers a unique opportunity to assess the functional potential of these cells in situ. The ISH technology is complex, depends on the availability of specific probes or oligonucleotides, and although it has been successfully used to study expression of mRNA for a variety of different cellular genes, its application to cytokine gene expression has been rather difficult. In part, this may be because expression of cytokine genes is tightly regulated, and mRNA for cytokines is not abundant in most cells. The most sensitive ISH methods, utilizing ^{35}[S]-labeled probes have been employed with success[5,6] in our and other laboratories.[7] However, to be successful with ISH, degradation of mRNA following tissue harvest must be avoided at all cost. This means that human biopsy tissues must be snap-frozen in the OR immediately after dissection. ISH for cytokine genes on fixed paraffin embedded archival tissues has not been reliable, possibly because of RNA degradation during storage.

HISTOPATHOLOGIC EVALUATION OF TIL

A great deal of variability exists among different solid tumors, even within the same histopathologic type, in the distribution of MNC infiltrates.[1,8] In general, MNC are located around the tumor, surrounding it like a wreath, and in the tumor stroma.[1,8] In some tumors, MNC may also be found in the tumor parenchyma, i.e., between or in touch with the tumor cells. The presence of infiltrating MNC inside a nest of tumor cells and in touch with the cells themselves has been interpreted as evidence of the ability of some inflammatory cells to localize to the tumor and perhaps mediate antitumor effects.[9] The intensity of MNC infiltrates is equally variable from one tumor to another, regardless of the tumor histology. There are, however, certain notable exceptions. For example, human primary melanomas are almost always well infiltrated and the degree of infiltration has been reported to indicate good prognosis.[10,11] Human squamous cell carcinomas of the head and neck (SCCHN) often contain large MNC infiltrates in the tumor stroma (Fig. 1), and the presence as well as intensity of the infiltrates has been linked to improved survival in this group of patients.[12,13] In ovarian carcinoma, tumors of low-malignant potential contain relatively few MNC, while malignant ovarian carcinomas, whether serous or mucinous are often very well infiltrated.[14] Among breast carcinomas, those which produce and secrete mucins appear to be better infiltrated than those which do not.[5]

An argument could be made that if TIL represent antitumor effector cells, then local accumulations of such cells in the tumor stroma or parenchyma should be beneficial to the host, and more intensely infiltrated tumors should have a better prognosis than poorly infiltrated ones. With few exceptions, however, it has not been possible to make this type of a correlation between TIL in the tumor and prognosis, even for histologically identical tumors. In reviewing the considerable literature on this subject that has accumulated over the last 30 years, three contradictory conclusions stand out: (a) the intensity of tumor MNC infiltrates correlates well with a better prognosis; (b) there is no evidence that the MNC infiltrate can be correlated with prognosis; and (c) a poor prognosis is associated with the presence of intense inflammatory infiltrates.[15] There may be several reasons for this lack of agreement among the data available. Most human tumors are in advanced stages by the time they come to surgery, and it is possible that TIL infiltrations observed at the time of biopsy may be different from those present during early disease not only in the intensity but also in composition of infiltrating MNC. Also, TIL which have remained in the tumor for a period of time are likely to be influenced by the tumor and various immunoinhibitory factors known to be produced by human tumors.[8] But most important is the fact that careful prospective studies with long follow-up are necessary to seek the correlation between the degree of infiltration and prognosis or survival, and such studies have not been done. Most studies found in the literature were retrospective.

Two recent reports have provided evidence that a poor prognosis is associated with a marked lymphoplasmacytic infiltration of the tumor.[16,17] In diffuse sclerosing papillary carcinoma of the thyroid[16] and in RCC,[17] the extent of lymphocyte infiltration of the tumor was quantitated and positively correlated with factors defining poor prognosis. Similar findings were described in breast cancer by Rosen[18] and Pupa et al.[19] The authors of these publications suggest that T cells infiltrating the tumor were responsible for stimulation of tumor growth. Concrete evidence that another human tumor can be stimulated by growth factors released by $CD4^+$ T lymphocytes comes from the group of Gallo et al[20] in a study of a long-term culture of Kaposi's sarcoma cells in vitro. The ability of TIL to facilitate tumor growth, at least in some tumors, has to be seriously considered in view of rapidly accumulating evidence that TIL are a source of multiple cytokines, many of which may have growth potentiating properties for tissue cells.[21,22] In addition, newer evidence indicates that tumor cells express receptors for cytokines[23,24] and that their growth may be either inhibited[23] or stimulated[25] by cytokines in the tumor microenvironment. These observations emphasize the fact that immune reactivity may not always be a good thing and that tumors are capable of adapting and taking advantage of the immune cells by cleverly manipulating the immunoregulatory mechanisms.

IMMUNOHISTOLOGY OF TIL

Immunohistology has greatly contributed to phenotypic characterization of TIL subpopulations in situ.[1,8] The proportions of lymphocytes to monocytes and of various lymphoid subpopulations of TIL in the stroma and parenchyma have been determined in many tumors.[1,8] In spite of a large degree of individual variability, it has been possible to conclude that T ($CD3^+CD2^+$ TcR^+) lymphocytes are the main component of infiltrates,[1,8] although in many tumors, monocytes are also prominent.[26,27] B lymphocytes are rarely found with the exception of melanoma,[11] and natural killer (NK) cells may be present, but in relatively small numbers.[28] In the tumor stroma, the CD4/CD8 ratios tend to be higher than in the parenchyma, which means that in the parenchyma $CD8^+$ T cells are more likely to be found in close contact with tumor cells than $CD4^+$ T cells.[1,29] The latter are mainly seen in the stroma.[30] In addition, variable but often substantial numbers of T cells in the tumor appear to be activated, because they express HLA-DR Ags.[10,30,31] On the other hand, $CD25^+$ T cells are less frequently found among TIL than are HLA-DR^+ cells,[32] although proportions of $CD25^+$ T cells are generally higher in TIL than in autologous PBL (A-PBL).[33] It is important to realize that

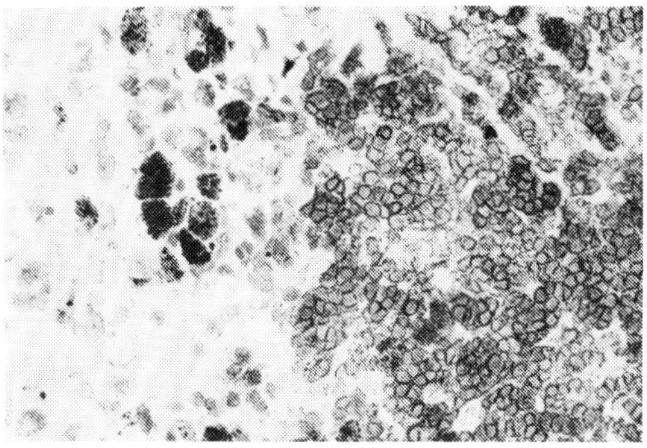

Fig. 4. Immunohistology of tumor-infiltrating lymphocytes (TIL) in cryostat tissue sections of malignant melanoma. Note the intense infiltrate of CD3⁺ T lymphocytes (right) next to tumor cells, some of which are strongly pigmented (left). Mag x 500.

the above conclusions do not apply to every solid tumor but represent a consensus derived from many different immunohistologic studies. Some of these studies are briefly highlighted below. The photomicrographs, which are used to illustrate TIL immunohistology in various human tumors, were taken in the author's laboratory (Figs. 2 to 9).

Immunohistology of Melanoma

Using an avidin/biotin immunoperoxidase system with mAbs to lymphocyte subsets, a number of investigators have studied the host response to malignant melanoma and melanocytic nevi in frozen sections.[10,11,34] The lymphocytic response to malignant melanoma and dysplastic nevi consists primarily of T cells (Fig.4), including both the CD4 helper/inducer and CD8 cytotoxic/suppressor phenotypes.[10,11,34] In addition, macrophages are also a prominent component of these lesions, as illustrated in Figure 2. Progression of human melanoma has been reported to be associated with changes in the phenotype of tumor cells.[34] During this progression, changes in localization, composition and activation state of the infiltrates were observed.[34,35] These changes included the decreased number of peritumoral T cells and of IL-2R$^+$ T cells as well as T6$^+$ (CD1a$^+$) dendritic cells.[35] In melanoma metastases, only scanty infiltrating cells were present.[35] The available data suggest that progression and metastatic spread of melanoma is associated with a decrease in the intensity of lymphocytic infiltrates. However, the pattern of TIL infiltrates is not a simple or direct prognostic parameter in melanoma, because metastatic tumors may be observed in the presence of a strong infiltrate within the tumor.[34,35]

Immunohistology of Breast Carcinoma

Many mammary carcinomas are infiltrated by MNC (Fig. 2), and the presence of these infiltrates has been interpreted as a favorable prognostic sign by some investigators.[15] In other studies, however, the prognostic significance of tumor infiltrates could not be confirmed.[15] While some studies show a predominance of CD4$^+$ T cells in breast tumors,[36,37] others show that CD8$^+$ T cells are more numerous.[38,39] Table 1 shows the results of immunohistologic analyses of 12 breast carcinomas performed in our laboratory.[40] The CD4/CD8 ratios varied from tumor to tumor, although in 8/12 breast tumors studied, CD8$^+$ cells were more numerous than CD4$^+$ lymphocytes. An interesting finding has been an inverse correlation of the degree of lymphocytic infiltrate, which was not related to tumor stage or histologic grade, with the level of estrogen receptors (ER) found within the tumor.[41] Again, others were unable to confirm this inverse correlation.[42]

Breast carcinomas are mucin-producing tumors, and the intensity of MNC infiltrates into the tumor has been related to the presence of mucin. Mucin-producing tumors are thought to induce strong immune responses and contain large MNC infiltrates (see also Fig. 5).[5,43] In another small series of breast tumors (n=13) studied in our laboratory, a degree of MNC infiltration, as determined by histopathology, was correlated with expression of mucins inside the tumor cells or in the lumen of ducts, using mucicarmine-stained sections.[5] As Table 2 indicates, in 12 cases of invasive ductal breast carcinoma and one case of cystosarcoma phylloides examined, there appeared to be no correlation between the intensity of inflammatory infiltrate and the presence of mucins. In 6/13 cases few tumor-infiltrating MNC were

Table 1. Histopathological diagnoses and immunohistology of human breast carcinomas studied

Histopathological diagnosis		Immunohistology					
		CD2⁺	CD4⁺	CD8⁺	CD15⁺	CD20⁺	Ratio CD4/CD8
		(cell counts in tumor stroma per 50 mm²ᵃ					
Patients without axillary metastasis:							
1. Infiltrating ductal CA		1040	600	360	52	40	1.67
2. Infiltrating ductal CA		190	144	64	0	0	2.25
3. Infiltrating ductal CA		1120	378	739	0	10	0.51
4. Infiltrating ductal CA		2360	900	1440	125	25	0.63
	mean	1178	506	650	44	19	1.27
	(±SE)	(±447)	(±161)	(±297)	(±28)	(±9)	(±0.4)
Patients with axillary metastasis							
1. Infiltrating ductal CA		145	49	90	0	36	0.55
2. Infiltrating ductal CA		1710	630	1170	0	57	0.54
3. Medullary CA		5100	2085	2800	0	240	0.74
4. Infiltrating ductal CA		953	130	754	0	18	0.17
5. Infiltrating lobular CA		160	45	109	0	16	0.41
6. Infiltrating ductal CA		185	70	136	14	22	0.51
7. Infiltrating ductal CA		2140	1488	620	20	126	2.4
8. Infiltrating ductal CA		1290	986	319	7	15	3.1
	mean	1460	685	750	5	66	1.05
	(±SE)	(±590)	(±277)	(±325)	(±2.8)	(±28)	(±0.4)

[a] Positively stained cells were counted in serial cryostat sections. Each section was stained with a different mAb.
(From Whiteside et al, Cancer Immunol Immunother 1986;23:169-178)

observed within the tumor. In the other 7 cases, large numbers of MNC were present in the stroma. In 5/9 tumors which contained ductal carcinoma in situ (DCIS), large infiltrates of MNC were present around the ducts involved in neoplastic proliferation (Fig. 5).

In a recently completed retrospective study of 1,200 cases of breast cancer, overexpression of the C-erb B2 oncogene was found to indicate a bad prognosis in the node-negative patients.[44] The oncogene overexpression was strongly correlated with the presence of lymphocytic infiltration in the tumor ($p=10^{-6}$). Thus, in this study, the presence of lymphocytes in the tumor was significantly associated with a poor prognostic factor.[44]

Immunohistology of Head and Neck Tumors

Primary SCCHN are generally well infiltrated with T lymphocytes.[12,13] In contrast, non-squamous-cell head and neck tumors appear to be poorly infiltrated with MNC.[31] In SCCHN, increased numbers of TILs around and in the tumor have been related to improved prognosis and survival.[12] Thus, in SCCHN, there exists preliminary evidence for involvement of TILs in the local immune response to tumor and in tumor regression.[12] In one of our own studies, including 16 cases of HNC, the tumors studied by immunohistology were well or moderately-well infiltrated with MNC (Fig. 6a). In the tumor

Table 2. Inflammatory infiltrate and the presence of mucins in human invasive breast cancer [a]

Case type	Histologic	DCIS	Infiltrate	Mucins
1.	IDC	+	+	I+
2.	IDC	+	2+	–
3.	IDC	2+	3+	–
4.	IDC	–	+	I/L 2+
5.	IDC	–	+	I/L +
6.	IDC	+	+	–
7.	IDC	–	3+	–
8.	IDC	2+	3+	I/L 3+
9.	Tub IDC	3+	2+	I/L 3+
10.	IDC	+	3+	I/L 3+
11.	IDC	+	+	I+
12.	CySaPh	–	–	–
13.	PAP IDC	3+	3+	I/L 3+

[a] Mononuclear cell infiltrates in the tumors were graded on histologic H&E-stained sections (– = negative; 1+ to 3+ positive), using a grading scale based on the average number of MNC per high power field (mag x 400) as follows: +, 10–30 cells; 2+, 30–50 cells; 3+, >50 cells. The presence of mucins inside tumor cells (I) in the lumen (L) of ducts was semi-quantified by two pathologists examining mucicarmine-stained sections. Abbreviations used are as follows: IDC = invasive duct carcinoma; Tub = tubular type; PAP = papillary type; CySaPh = cystosarcoma phylloides; DCIS = ductal carcinoma in situ.
(From Vitolo et al, Int J Cancer 1992;51:573-580)

stroma, infiltrates graded 4+ (i.e., containing greater than 250 MNC per 1 HPF at mag x 400) were present in 4 cases. Few MNC were seen in tumor parenchyma (Fig. 6b). The degree of infiltration with MNC in HNC did not correlate with extracapsular spread or tumor differentiation, and no correlations with prognosis were made because of a limited follow-up time (<16 months). Figure 6 c-f shows examples of the immunohistochemically stained MNC infiltrates found in primary SCCHN. $CD2^+$ and $CD3^+$ lymphocytes were the predominant populations infiltrating SCCHN, and as indicated in Figure 6, the intensity of lymphocytic infiltrates was highly variable, ranging from 1+ to 4+. Cells expressing an NK phenotype ($CD56^+$,$B73.1^+$, or $CD57^+$) were rare as were $CD15^+$ and IL-$2R^+$ cells. These tumors contained 30-50% of HLA-DR^+ and $CD71^+$ (transferrin-receptor) MNC. The double-staining immunoperoxidase method performed with anti-CD2 and -HLA-DR or anti-CD2 and -CD71 mAbs applied to the same sections of tumor tissue in selected cases indicated that activated T lymphocytes (i.e., T lymphocytes simultaneously expressing the CD2 and HLA-DR or CD71 Ags) were numerous in SCCHN (Fig. 3a). The mean CD4/CD8 ratio in tumor stroma was 2.4. In tumor

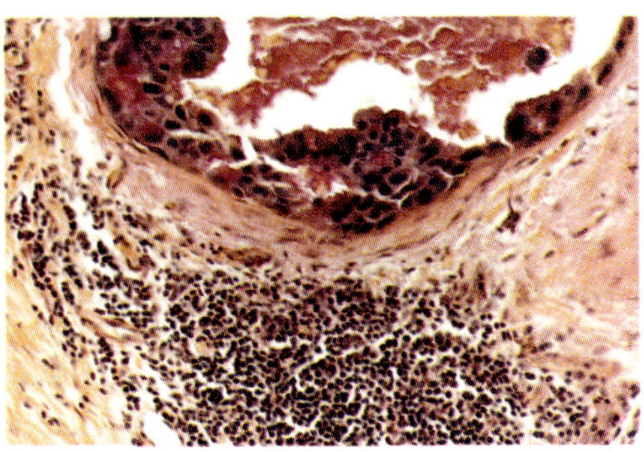

Fig. 5. A paraffin section of a mucin-producing breast carcinoma stained with mucicarmine. Note the presence of intracellular as well as extracellular mucin (red) and the heavy periductal infiltrate of MNC cells. Mag x 225. Reproduced with permission from Vitolo et al, Eur J Cancer, 1993;29:371-377.

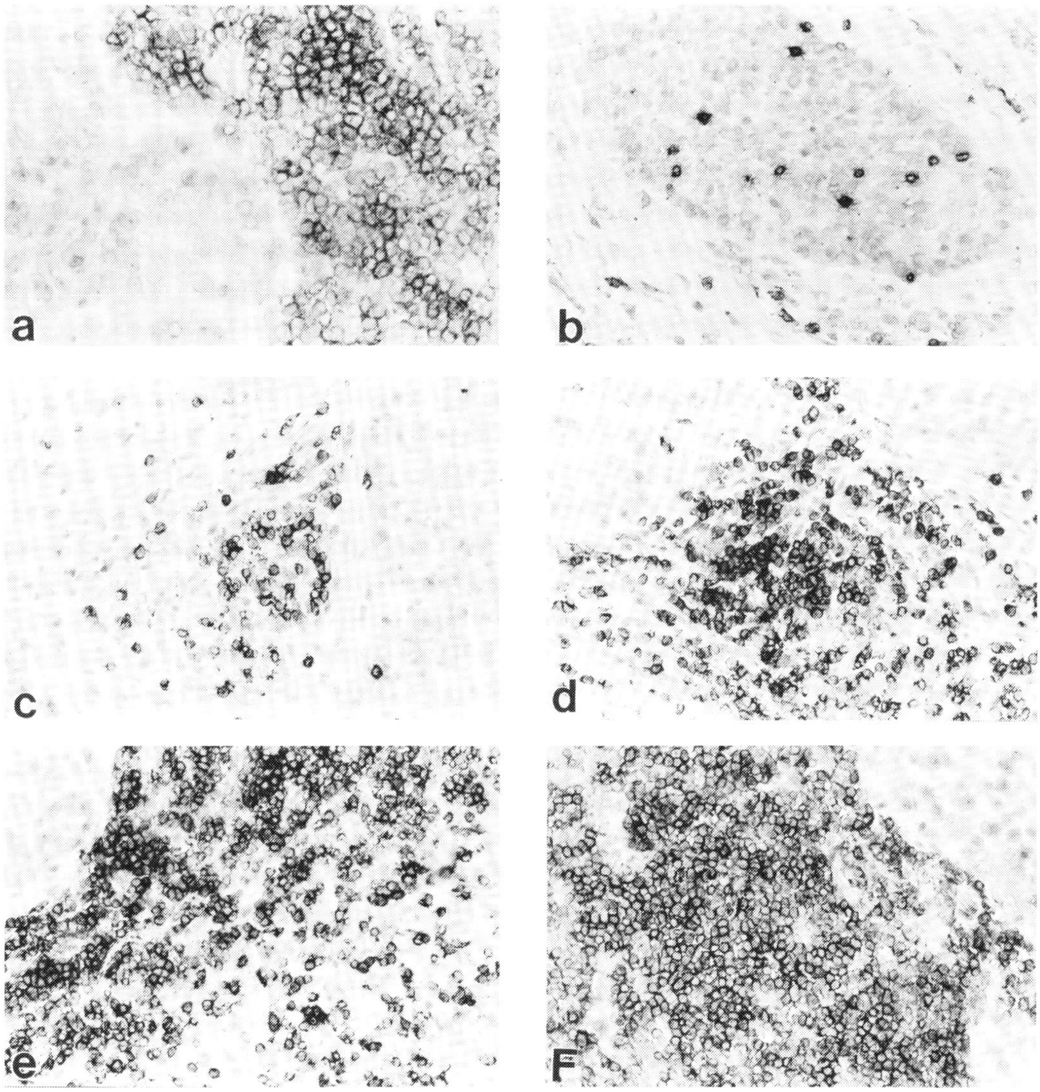

Fig. 6. Immunohistology of tumor-infiltrating lymphocytes (TIL) in cryostat sections of squamous cell carcinomas of the head and neck (SCCHN). In a, anti-CD3 mAb was used to demonstrate accumulation of T cells in the tumor stroma. In b, cells stained with anti-CD8 mAb in the tumor parenchyma. In c to d, various degrees of infiltration with $CD3^+$ T cells in SCCHN as follows: 1+ (c); 2+ (d); 3+ (e); and 4+ (f). Mag x 500. Reproduced with permission from Heo et al, Cancer Res 1987;47:6353-6362.

parenchyma, where $CD8^+$ cells always predominated, the CD4/CD8 ratio was 0.6 ($p<0.05$). In another study of 28 cases of SCCHN, we observed that tumor infiltrates were smaller in 3 patients with metastatic disease and 3 with recurrent tumors than in patients with primary SCCHN.[45] Overall, these and other immunohistologic studies of head and neck cancers (HNC) have indicated that TIL may play an active role in tumor progression, and that the host's ability to control tumor growth may, in part, depend on functional competence of these cells.

Immunohistology of Ovarian Tumors

The number and localization of TIL in normal ovarian tissue, ovarian tumors of low malignant potential (LMP) and invasive ovarian carcinoma were recently compared using immunohistology in our laboratory.[14]

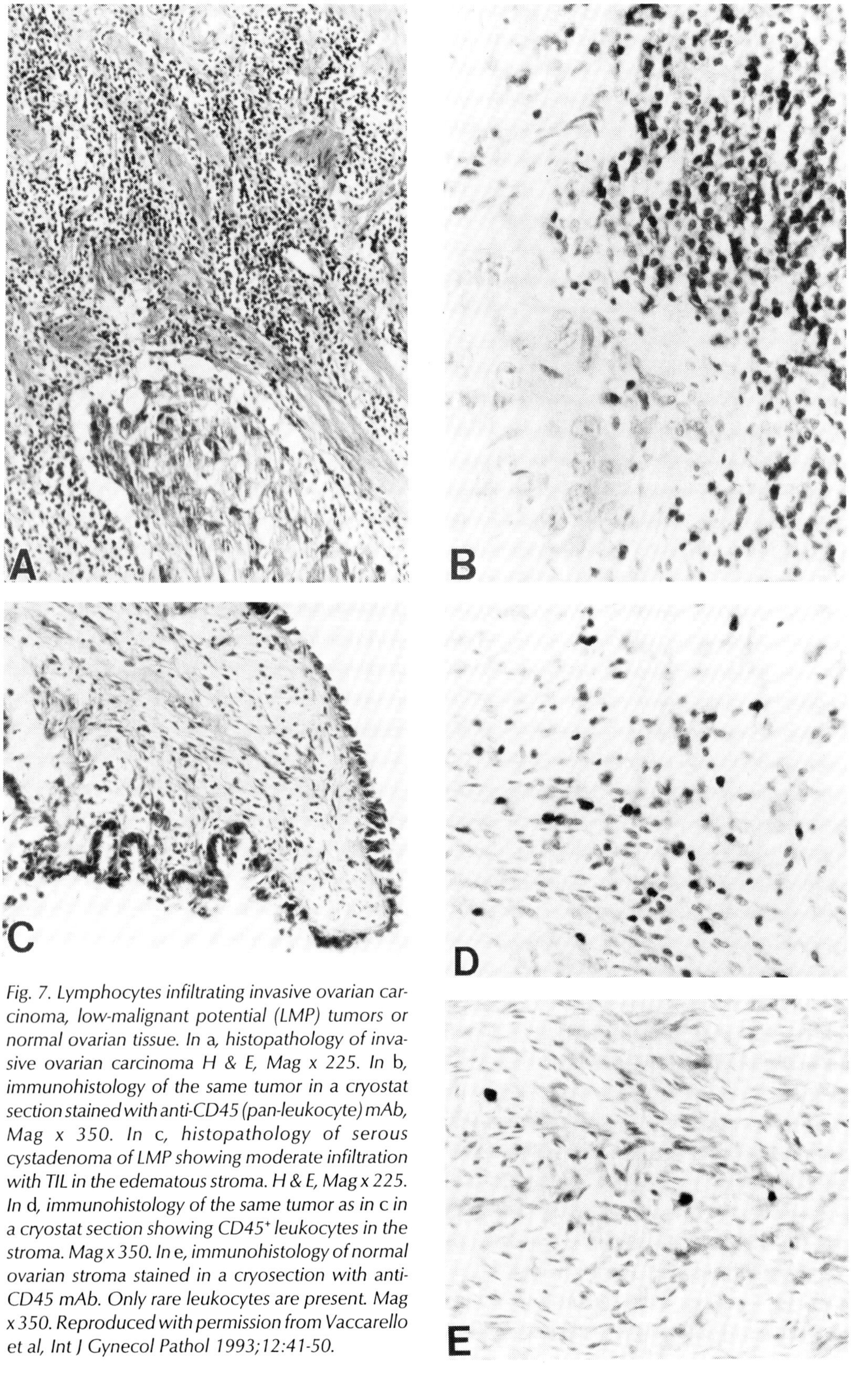

Fig. 7. Lymphocytes infiltrating invasive ovarian carcinoma, low-malignant potential (LMP) tumors or normal ovarian tissue. In a, histopathology of invasive ovarian carcinoma H & E, Mag x 225. In b, immunohistology of the same tumor in a cryostat section stained with anti-CD45 (pan-leukocyte) mAb, Mag x 350. In c, histopathology of serous cystadenoma of LMP showing moderate infiltration with TIL in the edematous stroma. H & E, Mag x 225. In d, immunohistology of the same tumor as in c in a cryostat section showing CD45^{+} leukocytes in the stroma. Mag x 350. In e, immunohistology of normal ovarian stroma stained in a cryosection with anti-CD45 mAb. Only rare leukocytes are present. Mag x 350. Reproduced with permission from Vaccarello et al, Int J Gynecol Pathol 1993;12:41-50.

Lymphocytes in normal ovaries were few in number and present mainly in the perivascular location and in corpora albican. Occasional lymphocytes were present in the ovarian stroma (Fig. 7a). In the serous LMP, TIL were +1 to +2/HPF and present mainly in the edematous stroma and in perivascular location (Figs. 7b,c). Few TIL also infiltrated the epithelium. In the mucinous LMP, TIL were +2/HPF in the stroma, especially in perivascular areas, and were enmeshed within the epithelium and in the mucinous secretion (Figs. 7d,e). The mixed LMP were similar to the mucinous LMP but contained fewer TIL within the epithelium. TIL were more numerous in the invasive ovarian CA (+4/HPF in Table 3). The greatest number of TIL were seen in the stroma; however, a fair number were located in the epithelium as well as in the secretion and in the necrotic portion of the tumor (Table 3 and Figs. 7d,e). Our finding that LMP ovarian tumors, which might be considered preinvasive lesions, contain more prominent infiltrates than those seen in normal ovarian tissues suggests the presence of more vigorous local immune response in these lesions.

Immunohistology of Colon Tumors

A large number of studies describing the in situ phenotype and distribution of TIL in colon tumors have been published.[1,46-48] Some of the more recent studies utilized video image analysis to obtain more accurate and objective results.[49] In one such study, the mean total number of MNC per mm^2 in histologically normal areas of the tissue was significantly higher than that in tumors themselves.[50] Stage A tumors had significantly higher numbers of MNC than stage B ($p<0.01$), C ($p<0.001$), and D ($p<0.001$) tumors. Well differentiated adenocarcinomas had a higher ($p<0.025$) density of MNC than poorly differentiated tumors. T lymphocytes formed the majority of TIL, with $CD4^+$ subset predominating in all except in 2/29 cases examined.[50] All sections of normal colon (4–6 cm distal to the tumor) also had more $CD4^+$ than $CD8^+$ cells. The proportion of $CD3^+$ cells in tumors was significantly higher than that in normal colon despite the overall reduction in MNC. In contrast to other reports,[47] few macrophages were present in either tumor or normal tissue, and B as well as NK cells were not detected.[41,46] This study

Table 3. Location and intensity of infiltrating cells positive for the leukocyte common antigen in normal ovarian tissue, tumors of low malignant potential, and invasive ovarian carcinoma[a]

	Infiltrating lymphocytes	Stroma	Epithelium	Secretion
Normal (n=4)	<+1	+1	-	-
LMP (n=7)				
Serous	+1 to +2	+1	<+1	-
Mixed SM	+1 to +2	+1 to +2	<+1	+1
Mucinous	+1 to +2	+1	+1	+1 to +2
Ovarian carcinoma (n=8)	+4	+4	+2 to +3	+2 to +3

[a] Immunohistology was performed and positive cells in the tumors or normal ovarian tissue were enumerated in one high power field (HPF). The grading scale was as follows: +1, <5 cells;+2, <10 cells; +3, <20 cells; +4, >20 cells/HPF. LMP = low malignant potential.
(From Vaccarello et al, Int J Gynecol Pathol 1993;12:41-50)

emphasizes an important point that immunohistology of tumor-uninvolved and normal tissues is necessary for meaningful interpretation of the TIL number and distribution in the colon as well as other organs or tissues. Figure 8 shows two examples of lymphocytic infiltrates seen in colon carcinomas in our laboratory.

Immunohistology of Primary Liver Tumors

Most human primary liver tumors do not contain impressive MNC infiltrates. The degree of infiltrates was generally scored as 1+ and rarely as 2+ in the tumor stroma.[32] Among one series of 16 hepatocellular carcinomas studied in the author's laboratory, there was one case with prominent T-cell

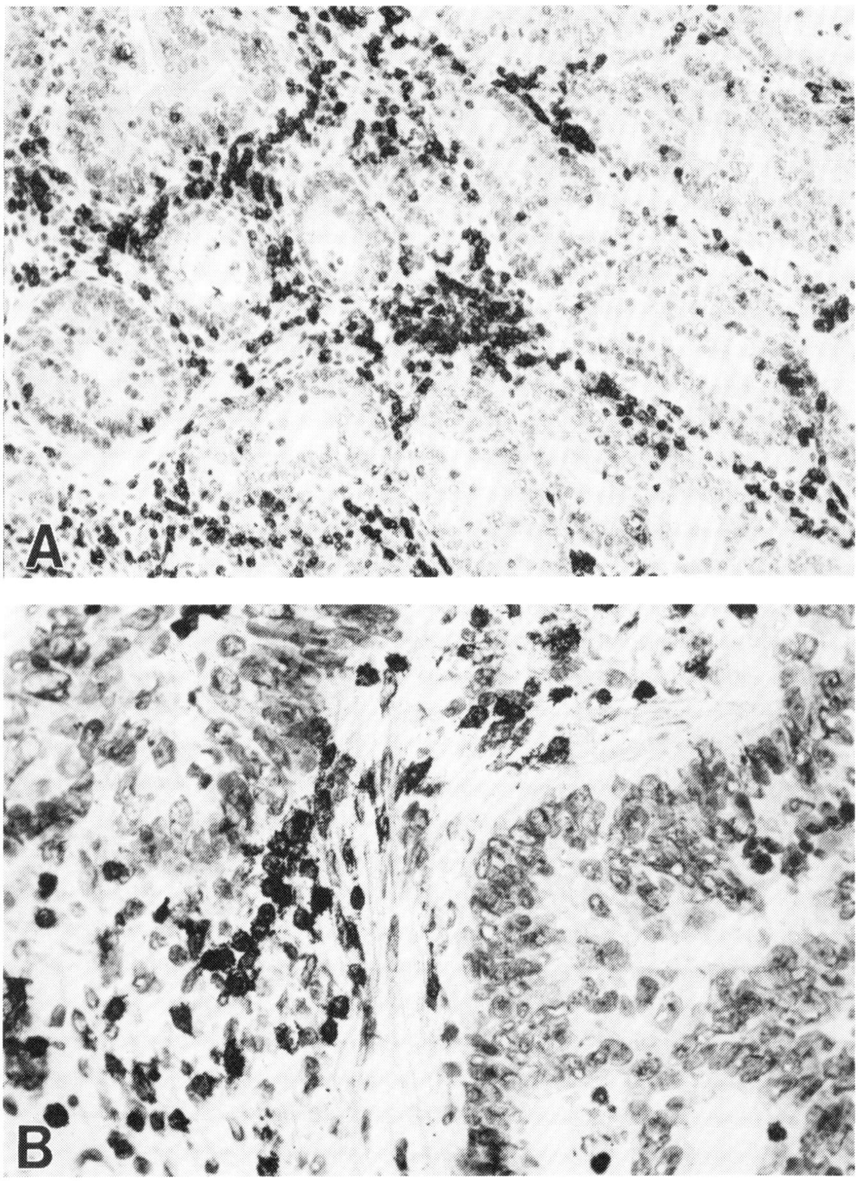

Fig. 8. Immunohistology of tumor-infiltrating lymphocytes (TIL) in cryostat sections of a colon carcinoma. In a, colon carcinoma stained with anti-CD3 mAb. Note CD3⁺ T lymphocytes in the tumor stroma. Mag x 130. In b, CD8⁺ T lymphocytes are seen in the tumor stroma and between tumor cells. Mag x 500. Figure 8b is reproduced with permission from Whiteside et al, Int J Cancer 1986;51:573-580.

infiltrates in the stroma (Fig. 9). Cholangiocarcinomas we studied were particularly poorly infiltrated with TIL. The helper/inducer T lymphocytes ($CD4^+$) predominated in the stroma and at tumor borders. In the parenchyma, tumor-infiltrating T cells in contact with tumor cells were few in numbers and tended to express the CD8 phenotype. The paucity of activated T lymphocytes (i.e., $HLA\text{-}DR^+$ or $IL\text{-}2R^+$), B-cells, NK cells, and $CD15^+$ cells in liver tumors was a consistent feature.[32] There were few differences between the primary and metastatic liver tumors in terms of the intensity or composition of mononuclear cell infiltrates. The only possible difference related to a near complete absence of NK cells and possibly a small increase in numbers of $CD15^+$ cells in metastatic liver tumors.[32]

Overall, immunohistology of solid tumors has contributed insights into the interactions between TIL and tumor cells, especially with regard to expression of the MHC Ags on tumor cells. In humans, the class I transplantation Ag is a 45 kD glycoprotein encoded by the A, B and C loci of the MHC and associated with a 12 kD β_2-microglobulin. The class II MHC Ag consists of a 34 kD α chain and a 28 kD β chain, and it is involved in the regulation of the immune response. While all nucleated cells express class I MHC Ags, class II MHC Ags appear mainly on B cells, macrophages, dendritic cells and other specialized cell types. Expression of the MHC Ags has been found to be altered in many tumor cells in comparison to normal cells.[51-54] These differences largely reflect quantitative but sometimes also qualitative modifications.[50,51,54] Attempts have been made to correlate the expression of these Ags on tumor cells with the intensity of MNC infiltrates into the tumor. However, although some evidence supporting the presence of large MNC infiltrates enriched in $CD8^+$ T cells in tumors expressing class I MHC Ags has been provided,[55,56] associations between these parameters remain largely unconfirmed. For example, some studies have shown a relationship between the level of class I and class II HLA Ag expression in primary cutaneous melanoma lesions and the degree of lymphocytic peritumoral[57] and intratumoral infiltrate,[58] respectively. In cutaneous metastases of melanoma, Ferrone and colleagues have observed that the absence or poor expression of HLA Ags on tumor cells occurred in lesions with scarce or absent MNC infiltrate. In contrast, marked lymphocytic infiltrates were present in lesions where most tumor cells were strongly stained for the class I and class II MHC Ags.[55] Similar findings were reported also for primary cutaneous melanoma lesions.[58]

The more recent availability of mAbs to adhesion molecules on human lymphocytes has permitted evaluation by immunohistology of interactions in situ between TIL and vascular endothelial cells (EC) as well as of TIL and tumor cells. In an immunohistologic study of human lung and RCC, Zocchi and Poggi have reported that both the cell surface protein CD31 (PECAM) and vascular cell adhesion molecule-1 (VCAM-1) were strongly expressed on vascular endothelium at the tumor site.[59] Most EC in tumor vessels expressed ICAM-1, and ICAM-1 was also found in the stroma and on tumor cells.[60] The CD31 molecule was also detected on a greater proportion of TIL than A-PBL T lymphocytes, and the integrin α 4 (CDw49d) was present on more than one third of TIL.[59] More than 95% of TIL were $CD11a/CD18^+$ ($LFA\text{-}1^+$), and about 65% expressed L-selectin (LAM-1). These findings suggest that the coexpression of CD31 molecules by TIL and

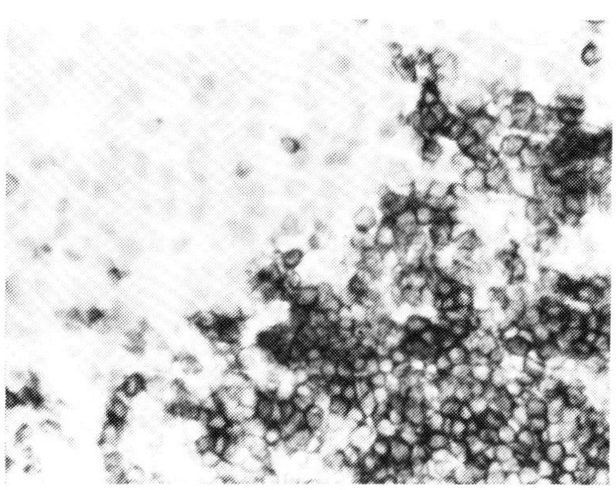

Fig. 9. Immunohistology of tumor-infiltrating lymphocytes (TIL) in a cryostat section of hepatocellular carcinoma. An intense infiltrate of $CD3^+$ T lymphocytes is present in this tumor. Mag x 550.

EC plays an important role in TIL-adhesion to EC at the tumor site. In addition, the LFA-1-ICAM-1 adhesion system is likely to be involved in TIL-tumor cell adhesion as well as TIL-EC interactions.[59]

As indicated by recent reports,[8,61] TIL are mainly T cells, which express the T cell receptor (TcR)α/β in most tumors, although, in some tumors, γ/δ^+ T cells may be present.[62] Immunohistology with mAbs to the V β chain of the TcR has been useful in confirming the oligoclonal nature of TIL in some human tumors.[63,64] Although the number of anti-human V β mAbs is still limited to only a few specificities, the use of these mAbs on cryostat tumor sections has been helpful in confirming molecular analyses of the V β gene restrictions in TIL in situ.[63,64]

Immunohistology has a number of limitations that have to be recognized. It is performed on fragments of tumor tissues especially sampled for this purpose, and its results cannot be generalized to the rest of tumor tissue, as local differences in composition (e.g., between the parenchyma and stroma; tumor periphery vs. interior) and intensity of infiltrates are known to exist. Certain lymphocyte surface Ags (e.g., the CD56 Ag) appear to be sensitive to air-drying and fixation necessary for immunostaining in situ, and no accurate information about the phenotype of cells expressing these Ags can be obtained.[65] As indicated earlier, immunohistology is also subjective, and a bias introduced by visual examination of serial sections, each stained with different mAb, has to be considered in interpreting results. Finally, while immunohistology characterizes TIL and tumor cells phenotypically and topographically, it offers no clues about their functional status.

Immunohistology can be and often is performed on paraffin rather than cryostat sections. In fact, paraffin sections offer a superior morphology and thus, a better, more precise way of defining the in situ spatial relationships between TIL and tumor cells. However, it is necessary to bear in mind that both fixation and tissue processing necessary for paraffin embedding might impair or alter the ability of certain Ags to react with mAbs. Thus, not only the sensitivity of Ag detection might be decreased following such processing, but certain Ags might become denatured. For these reasons, when immunohistology is performed with a given set of mAbs on paraffin sections, it is always advisable to simultaneously perform staining of cryostat sections of the same tissue to confirm that the relevant Ags are detected with comparable sensitivity. When performed and interpreted correctly, immunohistology is a very useful method, which has contributed greatly to a better understanding of the nature of MNC infiltrates present in or around human tumors.

IN SITU HYBRIDIZATION FOR CYTOKINE GENE EXPRESSION IN TIL

While histopathology and immunohistology provide information about location, distribution, intensity and phenotype of TIL, the state of their activation or function in the tumor environment might be, at least in part, evaluated using ISH for expression of cytokine genes. As recently demonstrated, cellular interactions are mediated by the cytokine network, consisting of soluble factors, cytokines, produced by activated cells and of receptors on target cells found in the tissue microenvironment.[66] Using ISH, it is now possible to determine expression of genes for various cytokines, for cytokine receptors and/or activation Ags in tissue. Since the tissue microenvironment determines, to a large extent, the types of signals that infiltrating MNC receive, expression of cytokine genes in TIL provides an estimate of their functional capabilities. Since TIL freshly isolated from a variety of tumors have been variously reported to be activated, functionally incompetent or enriched in antitumor effector cells, the possibility for determining functional capabilities of these cells in the tumor microenvironment is very important.

There are at least three different approaches to ISH for expression of cytokine genes. All three approaches require fresh tissues obtained from surgical biopsies. For successful ISH, it is essential that each tumor sample be snap-frozen in liquid nitrogen immediately after tumor dissection and stored at -80° for analysis by ISH and immunohistology. A portion of the same biopsy should also be fixed in formalin and processed for histology. In the first approach, the cDNA probes isolated from plasmids with respective restriction enzymes are used as the template for synthesis of antisense RNA as well as RNA sense probes, using T3 or T7 RNA polymerases. The probes are labeled with ^{35}[S] UTP (>1,000 Ci/mM). The labeled anti-sense RNA probe is used for hybridization with mRNA expressed in a cell.[7,67] The labeled sense probe is used as control and should give no positive signal. In the second approach, cDNA probes are labeled with ^{35}[S] dATP using a kit for random hexanucleotide priming, according to the method described by Feinberg and Vogelstein.[68] The specific activity of cDNA probes used for ISH has to be at least 1 x 10^8 cpm/µg of labeled fragment. The two strands of labeled cDNA probes are separated by boiling and the hybridization allowed to occur overnight in a humidified chamber at 45°C. In the third approach, ISH is performed using ^{35}[S] dATP-labeled oligonucleotides complementary to human cytokine mRNA. These oligonucleotides are labeled by using terminal deoxynucleotide transferase and purified by precipitation with 100% ethanol. In general, labeled antisense RNA probes or oligonucleotide probes are preferable, mainly because they provide a high level of specificity and low background. Also, the corresponding sense probes provide excellent negative controls. On the other hand, the use of cDNA probes has been quite successful in our hands. Although digoxigenin-labeled rather than ^{35}[S]-labeled probes are now available, they do not appear to be sensitive enough in our hands to consistently detect cytokine mRNA, and we have been more successful in using the ^{35}[S]-labeled probes. One disadvantage of this approach is that identification of the nature of cells which are positive is difficult, particularly in cryostat tissue sections, and a combination of ISH with immunohistology is necessary to precisely determine the nature of labeled cells. However, the combination of these two technologies is difficult and time consuming, particularly when applied to studies of cytokine mRNA. In most cells, these messages are present in low copy numbers and require both extremely carefully harvested tissues to avoid mRNA degradation and very sensitive techniques for detection. Positive controls for ISH in our hands include human peripheral blood MNC activated with 6,000 IU/ml of rIL-2 for three to five hours. In addition, tissue sections of normal "nonpathologic" specimens, such as tonsils, are routinely included. The presence of 18S ribosomal RNA is considered an indication that cells are synthesizing RNA, and this probe is always used as a positive control. Negative controls include cytosmears of resting MNC or tissue sections hybridized with ^{35}[S]-labeled pUC9 plasmid cDNA or with labeled sense probes, when RNA or oligo probes are used.

Using ISH in a recent study, we looked for expression of cytokine and IL-2R genes on serial cryostat sections of various human tumor tissues to determine if infiltrating MNC were activated, as judged by their ability to up-regulate gene transcripts for cytokines in the tumor microenvironment.[5,6] Human solid tumors used in this study included those prominently infiltrated with MNC as well as those containing sparse MNC infiltrates, as determined histologically. The proportions of TIL expressing genes for cytokines in ovarian adenocarcinoma, invasive breast cancer and SCCHN were determined. The invasive ductal breast carcinomas examined were divided into two groups based on the presence of MNC infiltrates in the tumor stroma. The tumors which produced large amounts of intraluminal or intracellular mucin, as determined by the mucicarmine stain, also contained large numbers of infiltrating MNC (Fig. 5). Among these MNC, from 18 to 30% contained gene transcripts for different cytokines and IL-2R (Fig. 10). In contrast, breast tumors which produced no or little mucins were poorly infiltrated with MNC (Table 4), and only rare MNC expressing cytokine genes (IL-2 and tumor necrosis factor [TNF]-α) were present.[5,6] No MNC expressing mRNA for IL-2R-α or -β were detected in these tumors. These results suggest that the ability of breast tumors to

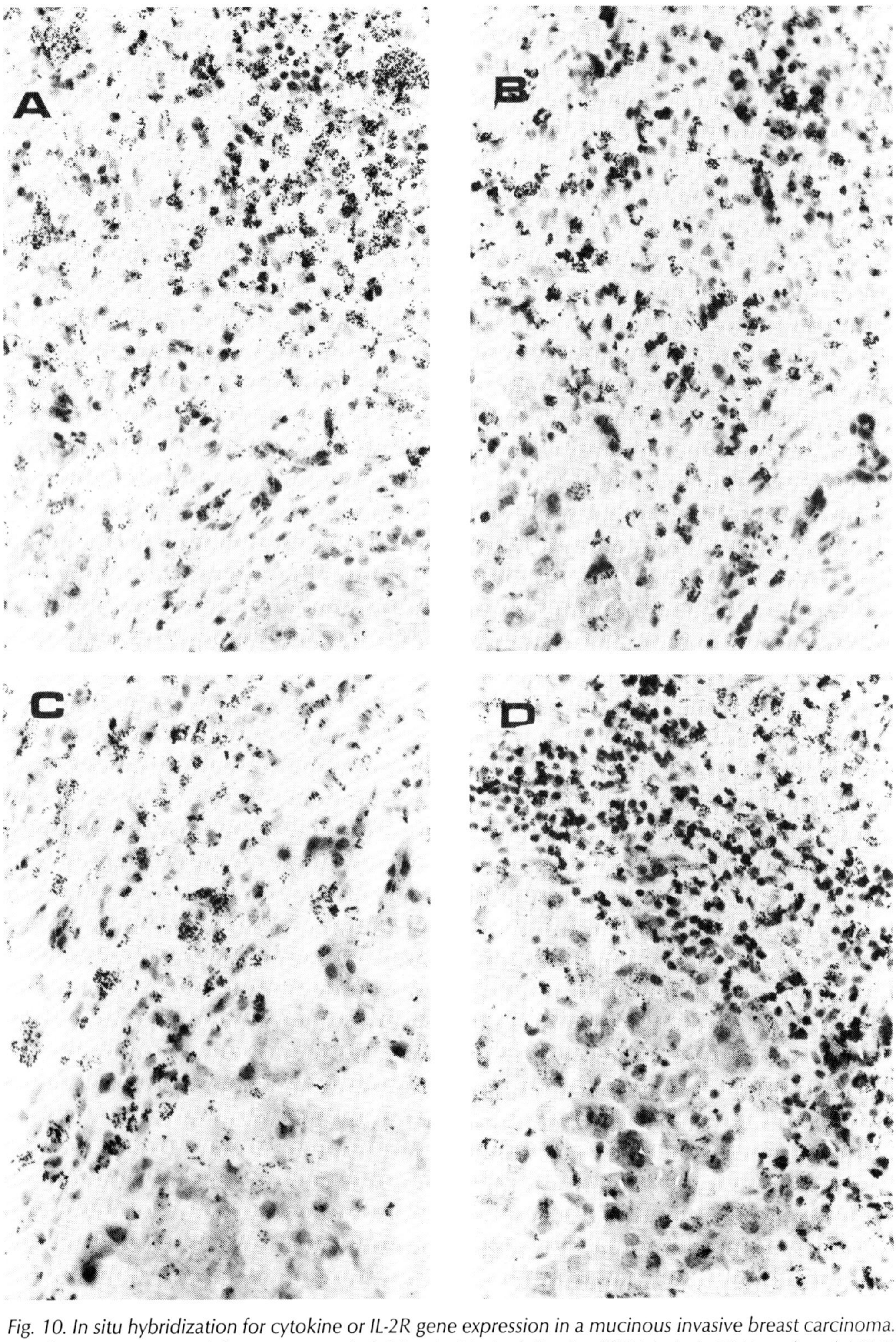

Fig. 10. In situ hybridization for cytokine or IL-2R gene expression in a mucinous invasive breast carcinoma. Serial cryostat section of the tumor were hybridized with the following ^{35}[S]-labeled cDNA probes: (a) TNF-α; (b) IFN-γ; (c) IL-2; and (d) IL-2R-α. Mag x 300. Reproduced with permission from Vitolo et al, Int J Cancer 1992;51:573-580.

Table 4. Expression of mRNA for cytokines or IL-2R by TIL in situ in human invasive breast carcinomas as determined by in situ hybridization[a]

Histology	n	TNF-α	IL-2	IFN-γ	IL-2R-α	IL-2R-β
		% positive cells				
Ductal; mucin-	9	1.2±1.6	0.9±1	0	0	0
Ductal; mucin+	4	23±5	4±8	21±15	23±6	15±8

[a] The data are means ± SD. Positive cells per 200 MNC were counted on serial tissue sections, each hybridized with a different ^{35}[S]-labeled cDNA probe. Positive cells contained >20 radioactive grains. Negative control slides did not contain radioactively-labeled cells. Positive control slides hybridized with 18S rRNA probe were 95-100% positive.
(Data are from Vitolo et al, Eur J Cancer 1993;3:371-377)

produce mucins may be associated with a more vigorous inflammatory or immune response, as compared to that seen in breast carcinomas which make little or no mucins.[5,6]

In contrast to breast carcinomas, only rare MNC expressing mRNA for cytokines were detected in the ovarian adenocarcinomas examined. Even in those ovarian tumors which were well infiltrated, only few cells positive for IL-2 (up to 5%) and IL-2R-α (up to 15%) were observed. No cells positive for interferon (IFN)-γ mRNA were detected in any of these tumors. All tumors contained a small proportion of MNC (up to 5%) expressing transcripts for tumor growth factor (TGF)-β.[5,6]

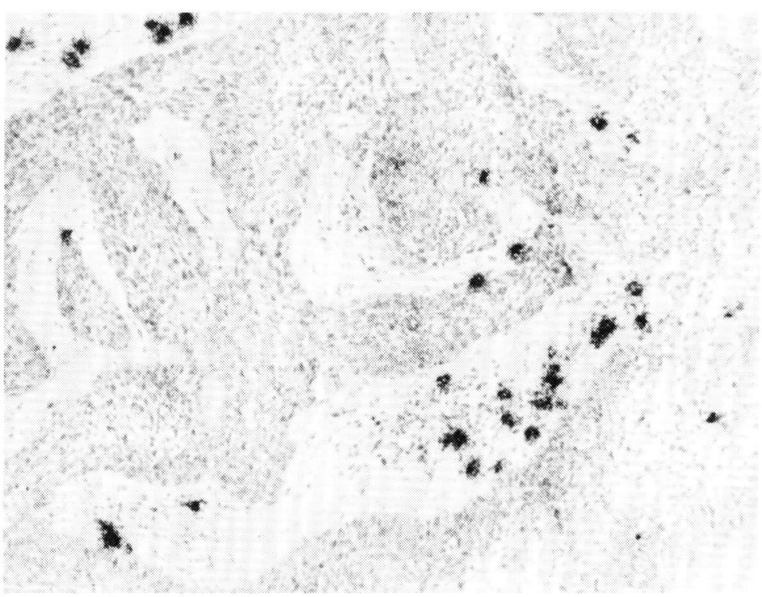

Fig. 11. In situ hybridization for cytokine gene expression in cryostat sections of SCCHN. ^{35}[S]-labeled cDNA probe for IL-2R-α was used for hybridization. Note positive cells in the tumor stroma. Mag x 125. Reproduced with permission from Vitolo et al, JNCI Monograph 1992;13:203-208.

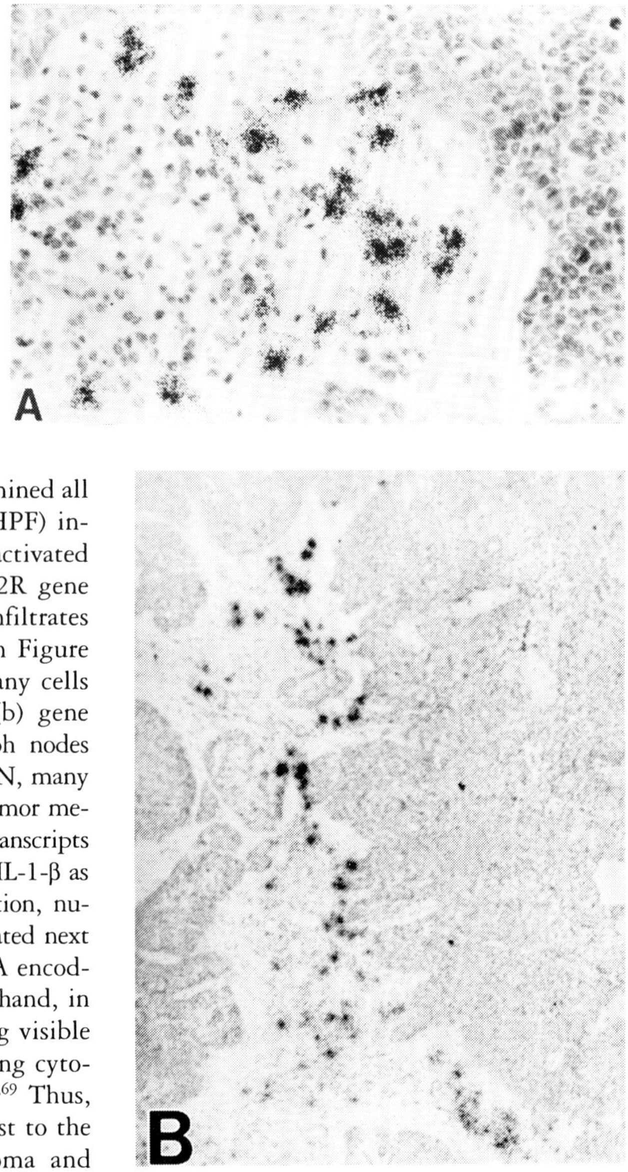

Fig. 12. In situ hybridization for cytokine gene expression in cryostat sections of SCCHN. In a, hybridization was performed with ^{35}[S]-labeled cDNA probe for TNF-α. Positive cells are in the tumor stroma. Mag x 400. In b, hybridization was performed with a probe for IFN-γ. Positive cells are in the tumor stroma, but in close proximity to the tumor cells. Mag x 100.

The three primary SCCHN examined all contained grade 2+ (30-50 MNC/HPF) infiltrates into the tumor stroma, and activated MNC positive for cytokine and IL-2R gene transcripts were present in these infiltrates (Fig. 11). For example, as shown in Figure 12, the tumor stroma contained many cells positive for IFN-γ (a) or TNF-α (b) gene transcripts. In tumor-involved lymph nodes obtained from 4 patients with SCCHN, many cells in an immediate proximity to tumor metastases were activated and contained transcripts for cytokines IL-2, IFN-γ, TNF-α or IL-1-β as well as for IL-2R-α or β.[6,69] In addition, numerous lymph node lymphocytes located next to tumor metastases contained mRNA encoding TGF-β (Fig. 13). On the other hand, in the lymph node areas not containing visible tumor metastases, few cells expressing cytokine or IL-2R genes were present.[6,69] Thus, it appeared that MNC located closest to the tumor, both in the SCCHN stroma and around metastases in the lymph nodes, were activated, while only few activated MNC were found in the tumor-uninvolved areas of lymph nodes.

In order to reliably utilize and correctly interpret the results of ISH for cytokine genes in human solid tumors, preliminary studies were necessary to examine cytokine mRNA expression in lymphoid cells populating normal human peripheral lymphoid tissues. Surprisingly, the number of cells expressing mRNA for cytokines was quite low in reactive lymphoid tissue in comparison to that in inflammatory nonlymphoid tissues examined.[5] Considerably higher numbers of cells positive for cytokine mRNA infiltrated chronic inflammatory tissues. This suggests that chronic antigenic stimulation might result in persistent cytokine mRNA expression and cytokine production. Therefore, we expected to find numerous cells positive for cytokines genes in human solid tumors containing TIL. Contrary to expectations, only a few randomly distributed MNC expressing mRNA for IL-2 were observed in the stroma of human ovarian carcinomas and of most nonmucinous invasive ductal breast tumors.

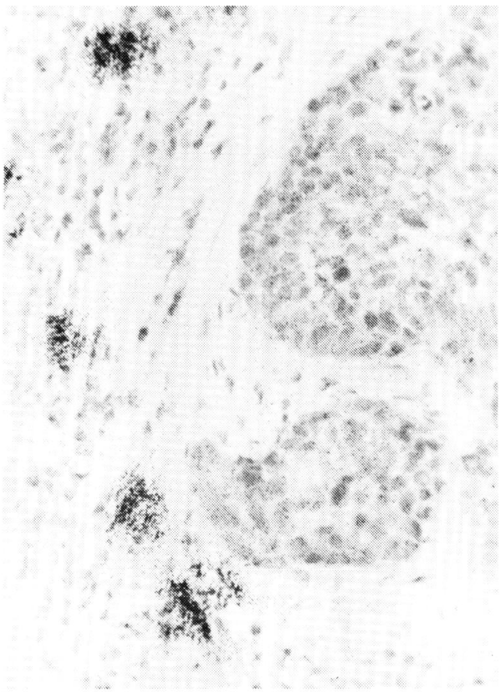

Fig. 13. In situ hybridization for cytokine gene expression. ^{35}[S]-labeled cDNA probe for TGF-β was used on a cryostat section of the tumor-involved lymph node from a patient with SCCHN. Mag x 400.

Our results indicated that various tumor types differed in the ability to modulate cytokine gene expression in infiltrating MNC. To a certain extent, this ability was related to the numbers of infiltrating MNC, in that MNC expressing cytokine or IL-2R gene transcripts were more numerous in well-infiltrated than in poorly infiltrated tumors. This observation is consistent with the hypothesis that tumor cells in certain, but not all solid tumors, can mediate recruitment of MNC and induce activation of infiltrating MNC.

It is also likely that the observed differences in expression of cytokine genes by TIL are related to the ability of tumor to activate MNC present in the local microenvironment on the one hand, and/or to down-regulate their function by delivering immunosuppressive signals on the other. We also obtained evidence that cells containing mRNA for TGF-β were frequently seen in SCCHN, and were present in small numbers in ovarian but not in breast carcinomas.[6] The localization of MNC containing TGF-β message in SCCHN or tumor-involved lymph nodes deserves attention. These MNC were found in the immediate proximity of tumor cells (see Figure 13) and were infrequent in tumor-uninvolved areas of lymph nodes. Thus, it appears that MNC activated by tumor-derived signals might express gene for TGF-β in addition to genes for other cytokines or IL-2R. In certain solid tumors, TGF-β producing MNC may be responsible for local regulation of antitumor responses and perhaps for local immunosuppression observed in in vitro experiments with freshly isolated TIL incubated with tumor cells.[70] Since interactions between TIL and tumor cells in the tumor microenvironment are probably mediated by cytokines, in situ studies of cytokine gene expression in either TIL or tumor cells or preferably both, provide important information about the cytokine circuits involved in the immunoregulation of tumor-infiltrating MNC functions in different types of human solid tumors.

Although mAbs to cytokines are available for immunohistologic detection of cytokines, this method does not adequately discriminate between the cytokine produced by a cell versus that occupying a cellular receptor. For this reason, we resorted to ISH for cytokine mRNA in lymphoid cells infiltrating solid tumors. The ability to identify and quantify in situ those TIL which express cytokine genes in the tumor is important for a better understanding of local events and for developing newer strategies for TIL activation. The method chosen for ISH using ^{35}[S]-labeled probes was found to be sensitive enough to detect mRNA for cytokines in single-cells as demonstrated in control experiments with peripheral blood MNC.[5,71]

Another new approach to in situ characterization of cytokine gene expression involves polymerase chain reaction (RT-PCR). Because of its exquisite sensitivity, RT-PCR can be used to probe for the presence of cytokine message in very few cells.[72] Unfortunately, it is not helpful in determining cytokine gene expression in TIL, simply because it is virtually impossible to separate TIL from tumor cells or tissue cells to the extent required for reproducible PCR. Since tumor cells as well as tissue cells might express messages for cytokines genes, contamination of TIL with either of these cell types makes RT-PCR impossible to interpret. For this reason, ISH is a technique of choice for determining cytokine gene expression in tissues. In addition to the presence of cytokine messages in individual cells, it is possible to also determine the localization of positive cells within the tissue, thus providing a map that might be useful for the analysis of tumor cell/TIL interactions in situ. For example, in a recently performed ISH study, it has been possible to demonstrate that IL-2 and IFN-γ mRNA were expressed in lymph node lymphocytes in low grade follicular lymphomas, and that these cytokine messages were expressed only in lymphocytes found in close contact with malignant cells.[7]

CYTOKINE PRODUCTION BY INDIVIDUAL CELLS IN THE TUMOR

While the presence of mRNA for cytokine genes in TIL or tumor cells generally implies that this message is translated into a protein, in pathologic situations, this assumption cannot be confidently made. The possibility of a posttranslational block has to be considered, especially with TIL, which are exposed to soluble factors produced and released by tumor cells. It is conceivable that some of these factors inhibit cytokine production. For this reason, it may be preferable to measure the ability of TIL to produce cytokines in situ. An assay for measuring cytokine release at the single-cell level, which also allows for immunophenotyping of individual cytokine-secreting cells in the population, has been described by Lewis.[73] The assay is basically a modification of the reverse hemolytic plaque assay (RHPA) established by Jerne many years ago.[74] Lewis has used the RHPA to visualize cytokine release by individual immunophenotyped infiltrating cells present in malignant human tumors.[75]

The RHPA is simple and cost effective. Briefly, it involves mixing of freshly isolated TIL preparations with an equal volume of ovine erythrocytes, which had been previously coupled to protein A. The mixture is placed in a Cunningham chamber to obtain a confluent monolayer of cells attached to the glass floor of the chamber. The chamber is then filled with an appropriate dilution of the antibody to a cytokine measured and, following an incubation period, guinea pig complement is added to initiate plaque formation. The area of hemolytic plaques formed is measured microscopically, using an image-analysis system. The cells in the center of plaques can then be visualized by immunohistology.[73,76]

Using this technique, Lewis and her collaborators studied secretion of IFN-γ and IL-4 by individual $CD16^+$ NK cells freshly isolated from either malignant tumor biopsies or peripheral blood of patients with ductal invasive breast cancer. Although NK cells are generally a minor component of TIL in most human tumors, it was possible to show, using the RHPA, that tumor-derived NK cells secreted more IFN-γ and IL-4 than those isolated from the blood of the same patients.[75] Thus, NK cells were induced to secrete these cytokines in the tumor microenvironment, possibly by tumor-derived signals, an observation similar to that reported by us for human purified NK cells incubated in the presence of SCCHN in vitro.[77]

This type of experimental approach allows for rapid and inexpensive screening of TIL freshly obtained from a tumor biopsy for the ability to produce cytokines spontaneously or following in vitro stimulation. Because of its simplicity, reliability and sensitivity, this assay seems to be applicable to verifying the results of ISH, which is a much more complex and difficult technique. In fact, this single-cell cytokine assay can be performed at the same time as ISH. A combination of molecular and functional in situ studies is clearly necessary to achieve an understanding of interactions between tumor cells and TIL in the tumor microenvironment.

A CRITICAL APPRAISAL OF IN SITU STUDIES WITH HUMAN TIL

Histologic, immunohistologic and more recent ISH or single-cell cytokine production studies of human TIL at the tumor site have resulted in significant advances. The majority of tumor-infiltrating MNC have been identified as $CD3^+TcR^+$ lymphocytes, although tumor-associated macrophages (TAM) are a substantial component of many tumor infiltrates. Immunohistologic characterization has confirmed that in most cases, T cells in tumor infiltrates express the TcR α/β, but in some tumors, notably in breast cancer and pulmonary cancers, TIL might express the TcR γ/δ.[58] Although only few mAbs specific for the different human TcR V β gene products are available, preliminary immunohistologic studies have suggested that TIL might be restricted in utilization of the TcR V β gene families. Using mAbs to activation Ags (e.g., anti-HLA-DR, anti-IL-2R, anti-CD71), it has been possible to confirm that TIL present in the tumor nests or even those in the tumor stroma frequently express activation Ags, although the proportion of T cells positive for these Ags varies widely even in tumors with the same histology. T cells found in tumors are mixtures of $CD8^+$ and $CD4^+$ cells, and it has not been possible to demonstrate that predominance of one or the other T-cell subpopulation in the tumor is in any consistent fashion related to better prognosis or survival. Most important, histopathologic and immunohistopathologic studies have not been able to confirm the early impression that the intensity of MNC infiltrates in the tumor is related to prognosis or survival. While this conclusion appears to be counter-intuitive, it emphasizes the fact that simply looking at cells at the tumor site is not adequate for deducing their biologic role in respect to tumor growth and progression. In this context, ISH for expression of cytokine genes or genes for cytokine receptors offers a broader definition of these cells, in that it provides information about their functional status in situ. It should be remembered that TIL as well as tumor cells may express mRNA for, and perhaps produce, a variety of cytokines which are likely to modulate the behavior of cells in the tumor microenvironment. Ultimately, it may not be the numbers or types of MNC in the tumor infiltrate but their ability to release cytokines or to mediate antitumor effects that will determine tumor progression or regression. The more recent data seem to indicate that the intensity or type of TIL infiltrates in human tumors may be related to characteristics of each individual tumor and its ability to modify the microenvironment. Among such characteristics, which might be particularly relevant to the state of TIL activation in situ, are the expression of immunogenic tumor-associated antigens (TAA) and the ability of the tumor to secrete immunosuppressive or immunostimulatory factors. These characteristics of the tumor, i.e., the capability to induce immunologic response in TIL, on the one hand, and to produce immunoinhibitory soluble factors, on the other, offer a plausible explanation for the observed lack of correlation between the intensity or cellular composition of tumor-infiltrating MNC and prognostic significance of these tumor infiltrates.

References

1. Vose BM, Moore M. Human tumor-infiltrating lymphocytes: A marker of host response. Semin Hematol 1985; 22:27-40.
2. Svennevig JL, Lunde OC, Holter J, Bjorgsvik D. Lymphoid infiltration and prognosis in colorectal carcinoma. Br J Cancer 1984; 49:375-377.
3. Hsu SM, Raine L, Fanger H. Use of avidin-biotin-peroxidase complex (ABC) in immunoperoxidase techniques: A comparison between ABC and unlabeled antibody (PAP) procedures. J Histochem Cytochem 1981; 29:577-580.
4. Chen K, Demetris AJ, Van Thiel DH, Whiteside TL. Double immunoenzyme staining method for analysis of tissue and blood lymphocyte subsets with monoclonal antibodies. Lab Invest 1987; 56:114-119.
5. Vitolo D, Zerbe T, Kanbour A, Dahl C, Herberman RB, Whiteside TL. Expression of mRNA for cytokines in tumor-infiltrating mononuclear cells in ovarian adenocarcinoma and invasive breast cancer. Int J Cancer 1992; 51:573-580.
6. Vitolo D, Kanbour A, Johnson JT, Herberman RB, Whiteside TL. In situ hybridization for cytokine gene transcripts in the solid tumor microenvironment. Eur J Cancer 1993; 3:371-377.
7. Peuchmaur M, Emilie D, Crevon M-C,

Brousse N, Gaulard P, D'Agay M-F, Galanaud P, Solal-Celigny P. Interleukin-2 and interferon-γ production in follicular lymphomas. Hematopathol 1991; 95:55-62.

8. Whiteside TL, Jost LM, Herberman RB. Tumor-infiltrating lymphocytes: Potential and limitations to their use for cancer therapy. Crit Rev Oncol /Hematol 1992; 25-47.
9. Paradis IL, Dauber JH, Rogers RM, Rabin BS. Lymphocyte subset distribution on the margins of lung cancers. Chest 1982; 82:234.
10. Poppema S, Brocker EB, de Leij L, Terbrack D, Visscher T, Ter Haar A, Macher E, The TH, Sorg C. In situ analysis of the mononuclear cell infiltrate in primary malignant melanoma of the skin. Clin Exp Immunol 1983; 51:77-82.
11. Kornstein MJ, Brooks JS, Elder DE. Immunoperoxidase localization of lymphocyte subsets in the host response to melanoma and nevi. Cancer Res 1983; 43:2749-2753.
12. Wolf GT, Hudson JL, Peterson KA, Miller HL, McClatchey KD. Lymphocyte subpopulations infiltrating squamous carcinomas of the head and neck: correlations with extent of tumor and prognosis. Otolaryngol Head Neck Surg 1986; 95:142-152.
13. Snyderman CH, Heo DS, Chen K, Whiteside TL, Johnson JT. T-cell markers in tumor-infiltrating lymphocytes of head and neck cancer. Head & Neck 1989; 11:331-336.
14. Vaccarello L, Kanbour A, Kanbour-Shakir A, Whiteside TL. Tumor-infiltrating lymphocytes from ovarian tumors of low malignant potential. Int J Gynecol Pathol 1993; 12:41-50.
15. Stewart THM, Tsai S-CJ. The possible role of stromal cell stimulation in worsening the prognosis of a subset of patients with breast cancer. Clin Expt Metastasis 1993; 11:295-305.
16. Gomez-Morales M, Alvaro T, Munoz Garcia Del Moral R, Aguilar D, Caballero T, Aneiros J. Diffuse sclerosing papillary carcinoma of the thyroid gland: Immunohistochemical analysis of the local host immune response. Histopathol 1991; 18:427-433.
17. Kolbeck PC, Kaveggia FF, Johansson SL, Grune MT, Taylor RJ. The relationships among tumor-infiltrating lymphocytes, histopathologic findings, and long-term clinical follow-up in renal cell carcinoma. Modern Pathol 1992; 5:420-425.
18. Rosen PP, Groshen S. Factors influencing survival and prognosis in early breast carcinoma: Assessment of 644 patients with median follow-up of 18 years. Surg Clin N Amer 1990; 70:937-962.
19. Pupa SM, Menard S, Andreola S, Rilke F, Cascinelli N, Colnaghi MI. Prognostic significance for C-erb B-2 oncoprotein overexpression in breast carcinoma patients and its immunological role. Proc AACR 1992; 33:312.
20. Nakamura S, Salahuddin SZ, Biberfeld P, Ensoli B, Markham PD, Wong-Staal F, Gallo RC. Kaposi's sarcoma cells: Long-term culture with growth factor from retrovirus-infected CD4+ T cells. Science 1988; 242:426-430.
21. Schwartzentruber DJ, Topalian SL, Mancini M, Rosenberg SA. Specific release of granulocyte-macrophage colony-stimulating factor, tumor necrosis factor-α, and IFN-γ by human tumor-infiltrating lymphocytes after autologous tumor stimulation. J Immunol 1991; 146:3674-3681.
22. Hom SS, Schwartzentruber DJ, Rosenberg SA, Topalian SL. Specific release of cytokines by lymphocytes infiltrating human melanomas in response to shared melanoma antigens. J Immunother 1993; 13:18-30.
23. Weidmann E, Sacchi M, Plaisance S, Heo DS, Yasumura S, Lin WC, Johnson JT, Herberman RB, Azzarone B, Whiteside TL. Receptors for interleukin 2 on human squamous cell carcinoma cell lines and tumor in situ. Cancer Res 1992; 52:5963-5970.
24. Morisaki T, Yuzuki DH, Lin RT, Foshag LJ, Morton DL, Hoon DSB. Interleukin 4 receptor expression and growth inhibition of gastric carcinoma cells by interleukin 4. Cancer Res 1992; 52:6059-6065.
25. Packard BS. Mitogenic stimulation of human tumor-infiltrating lymphocytes by secreted factor(s) from human tumor cell lines. PNAS USA 1990; 87:4058-4062.
26. Svennevig JL, Svaar H. Content and distribution of macrophages and lymphocytes in solid malignant human tumours. Int J Cancer 1979; 24:754-758.
27. Gottlinger HG, Rieber P, Gokel JM, Lohe

KJ, Riethmuller G. Infiltrating mononuclear cells in human breast carcinoma: Predominance of T4+ monocyte cells in the tumor stroma. Int J Cancer 1985; 35:199-205.
28. Introna M, Allavena P, Biondi A, Colombo N, Villa A, Mantovani A. Defective natural killer activity within human ovarian tumors: Low numbers of morphologically defined effectors present in situ. JNCI 1983; 70:21-26.
29. Cardi G, Mastrangelo MJ, Berd D. Depletion of T-cells with the CD4+CD45R+ phenotype in lymphocytes that infiltrate subcutaneous metastases of human melanoma. Cancer Res 1989; 49:6562-6565.
30. Whiteside TL, Heo DS, Chen K, Adler A, Johnson JT, Herberman RB. Expansion of tumor-infiltrating lymphocytes from human solid tumors in interleukin 2. In: Truitt RL, Gale RP, Bortin MM., eds.Cellular Immunotherapy of Cancer. New York, NY: Alan Liss, Inc., 1987: 213-222.
31. Heo DS, Whiteside TL, Johnson JT, Chen K, Barnes EL, Herberman RB. Long-term interleukin 2-dependent growth and cytotoxic activity of tumor-infiltrating lymphocytes (TIL) from human squamous cell carcinomas of the head and neck. Cancer Res 1987; 47:6353-6362.
32. Takagi S, Chen K, Schwarz R, Iwatsuki S, Herberman RB, Whiteside TL. Functional and phenotypic analysis of tumor-infiltrating lymphocytes isolated from human primary and metastatic liver tumors and cultured in recombinant interleukin 2. Cancer 1989; 63:102-111.
33. Whiteside TL, Heo DS, Takagi S, Herberman RB. Tumor-infiltrating lymphocytes from human solid tumors: Antigen-specific killer T lymphocytes or activated natural killer lymphocytes. In: Stevenson HC., ed.Adoptive Cellular Immunotherapy of Cancer. New York: Marcel Dekker, 1989: 139-157.
34. Brocker EB, Zwadlo G, Holzmann B, Macher E, Sorg C. Inflammatory cell infiltrates in human melanoma at different stages of tumor progression. Int J Cancer 1988; 41:562-567.
35. Brocker EB, Suter L, Bruggen J, Ruiter DJ, Macher E, Sorg C. Phenotypic dynamics of tumor progression in human malignant melanoma. Int J Cancer 1985; 36:29-35.
36. Whitwell HL, Hughes HPA, Moore M, Ahmed A. Expression of MHC antigens and leukocyte infiltration in benign and malignant human breast disease. Br J Cancer 1984; 49:161-172.
37. von Kleist S, Berling J, Bohle W, Wittekind C. Immunohistochemical analysis of lymphocyte subpopulations infiltrating breast carcinomas and benign lesions. Int J Cancer 1987; 40:18-23.
38. Bhan AK, Des Marais CL. Immunohistology characterization of major histocompatibility antigens and inflammatory cellular infiltrate in human breast cancer. JNCI 1983; 71:507-516.
39. Bilik R, Mor C, Hazaz B, Moroz C. Characterization of T-lymphocyte subpopulations infiltrating primary breast cancer. Cancer Immunol Immunother 1989; 28:143-147.
40. Whiteside TL, Miescher S, Hurlimann J, Moretta L, Von Fliedner V. Clonal analysis and in situ characterization of lymphocytes infiltrating human breast carcinomas. Cancer Immunol Immunother 1986; 23:169-178.
41. An T, Sood U, Pietruk T, Cummings G, Hashimoto K, Crissman JD. In situ quantitation of inflammatory mononuclear cells in ductal infiltrating breast carcinoma. Am J Pathol 1987; 128:52-60.
42. Underwood JCE, Giri DD, Rooney N, Lonsdale R. Immunophenotype of the lymphoid cell infiltrates in breast carcinomas of low estrogen receptor content. Br J Cancer 1987; 56:744-746.
43. Jerome KR, Barnd DL, Bendt KM, Bower CM, Taylor-Papadimitriou J, McKendzie IF, Bast Jr,R.C., Finn OJ. Cytotoxic T lymphocytes derived from patients with breast adenocarcinoma recognize an epitope present on the protein core of a mucin molecule preferentially expressed by malignant cells. Cancer Res 1991; 51:2908-2916.
44. Rilke F, Colnaghi MI, Cascinelli N, Andreola S, Baldini MT, Bufalino R, Della Porta G, Menard S, Pierotti MA, Testori A. Prognostic significance of HER-2/neu expression in breast cancer and its relationship to other prognostic factors. Int J Cancer 1991; 49:44-49.
45. Whiteside TL. Human tumor-infiltrating lymphocytes and their characterization. In:

Lotzova E, Herberman RB., eds.Role of Interleukin 2 Activated Killer Cells in Cancer. Boca Raton: CRC Press, Inc., 1990: 133-151.
46. Csiba A, Whitwell HL, Moore M. Distribution of histocompatibility and leukocyte differentiation antigens in normal human colon and in benign and malignant colonic neoplasms. Br J Cancer 1984; 50:699-709.
47. Allen C, Hogg N. Elevation of infiltrating mononuclear phagocytes in human colorectal tumors. JNCI 1987; 78:465-469.
48. Koch B, Giedl J, Hermanek P, Kalden JR. The analysis of mononuclear cell infiltrations in colorectal adenocarcinoma. J Cancer Res Clin Oncol 1985; 109:142-151.
49. Jarvis LR. Microcomputer video image analysis. J Microscopy 1987; 150:83-97.
50. Norazmi MN, Hohmann AW, Skinner JM, Jarvis LR, Bradley J. Density and phenotype of tumor-associated mononuclear cells in colonic carcinoma determined by computer-assisted video image analysis. Immunol 1990; 69:282-286.
51. Carrel S, Schmidt-Kessen A, Guiffre L. Recombinant interferon γ can induce the expression of HLA-DR and -DQ on DR-negative melanoma cells and enhance the expression of HLA ABC and tumor-associated antigens. Eur J Immunol 1985; 15:118-124.
52. Natali PG, Giacomini P, Bigotti K, Nicotra MR, Ng AK, Ferrone S. Heterogeneity in the expression of HLA and tumor-associated antigens by surgically removed and cultured breast carcinoma cells. Cancer Res 1983; 43:660-668.
53. Doyle A, Martin WJ, Funa K, Gazdar A, Carney D, Martin SE, Linnoila I, Cuttitta F, Mulshine J, Bunn P, Mina J. Markedly decreased expression of class histocompatibility antigens, protein, and mRNA in human small-cell lung cancer. J Exp Med 1985; 161:1135-1151.
54. Momburg F, Degener T, Bacchus E, Moldenhauer G, Hammerling GJ, Moller P. Loss of HLA-A, B, C and de novo expression of HLA-D in colorectal cancer. Int J Cancer 1986; 37:179-184.
55. van Duinen SG, Ruiter DJ, Brocker EB, van der Velde EA, Sorg C, Welvaart K, Ferrone S. Level of HLA antigens in locoregional metastasis and clinical course of the disease in patients with melanoma. Cancer Res 1988; 48:1091-1025.
56. Allen CA, Hogg N. Association of colorectal epithelium expression of HLAD/DR with CD8+ T cells and mononuclear phagocytes. Cancer Res 1987; 47:2919-2923.
57. Ruiter DJ, Bahn AK, Harrist TJ, Sorber AJ, Mihm Jr, M.C. Major histocompatibility antigens and mononuclear inflammatory infiltrate to benign nevo melanocytic proliferations and malignant melanoma. J Immunol 1982; 129:2808-2815.
58. Brocker EB, Suter L, Sorg C. HLA-DR antigen expression in primary melanomas of the skin. J Invest Dermatol 1984; 82:244-247.
59. Zocchi MR, Poggi A. Lymphocyte-endothelial cell adhesion molecules at the primary tumor site in human lung and renal cell carcinomas. JNCI 1993; 85:246-247.
60. Tomita Y, Nishiyama T, Watanabe H, Fujiwara M, Sato S. Expression of intercellular adhesion molecule-1 (ICAM-1) on renal cell cancer: Possible significance in host immune responses. Int J Cancer 1990; 46:1001-1006.
61. Ioannides CG, Whiteside TL. T-cell recognition of human tumors: Implications for molecular immunotherapy of cancer. Clin Immunol Immunopathol 1993; 66:91-106.
62. Zocchi MR, Ferrarini M, Rugarli C. Selective lysis of the autologous tumor by δ TCS1+ γ/δ+ tumor-infiltrating lymphocytes from human lung carcinomas. Eur J Immunol 1990; 20:2685-2689.
63. Janson CH, Grunewald J, Osterborg A, DerSimonian H, Brenner MB, Mellstedt H, Wigzell H. Predominant T-cell receptor V gene usage in patients with abnormal clones of B cells. Blood 1991; 77:1776-1780.
64. Jack AS, Boylston AW, Carrel S, Grigor I. Cutaneous T-cell lymphoma cells employ a restricted range of T-cell antigen receptor variable region genes. Am J Pathol 1990; 136:17-21.
65. Hata K, Zhang XR, Iwatsuki S, Van Thiel DH, Herberman RB, Whiteside TL. Isolation, phenotyping and functional analysis of lymphocytes from human liver. Clin Immunol Immunopathol 1990; 56:401-419.
66. Mantovani A, Dejana E. Cytokines as communication signals between leukocytes and

endothelial cells. Immunol Today 1990; 10:370-375.
67. Granelli-Piperno A. In situ hybridization for interleukin 2 and interleukin 2 receptor mRNA in T cells activated in the presence or absence of cyclosporin A. J Exp Med 1988; 168:1649-1658.
68. Feinberg AP, Vogelstein B. Addendum: A technique of radiolabelling DNA restriction endonuclease fragments to high-specific activity. Anal Biochem 1984; 137:266-267.
69. Vitolo D, Letessier EM, Johnson JT, Whiteside TL. Immunologic effector cells in head and neck cancer. In: Biology of and Novel Therapeutic Approaches for Epithelial Cancers of the Aerodigestive Tract. JNCI Monographs, 1992; 13:203-208.
70. Miescher S, Whiteside TL, Carrel S, Von Fliedner V. Functional properties of tumor-infiltrating and blood lymphocytes in patients with solid tumors: Effects of tumor cells and their supernatants on proliferative responses of lymphocytes. J Immunol 1986; 136:1899-1907.
71. Vitolo D, Vujanovic N, Rabinowich H, Schlesinger M, Herberman RB, Whiteside TL. Rapid interleukin-2 induced adherence of human natural killer (NK) cells: II. Expression of mRNA for cytokines and IL-2 receptors in adherent NK cells. J Immunol 1993; In press.
72. Legoux P, Minty C, Delpech B, Minty AJ, Shire D. Simultaneous quantitation of cytokine mRNAs in interleukin-1 β stimulated U373 human astrocytoma cells by a polymerization chain reaction method involving co-amplification with an internal multi-specific control. Eur Cytokine Netw 1992; 3:553-563.
73. Lewis CE. Cytokine production by individual cells. In: Balkwill FR., ed.Cytokines: A Practical Approach. Oxford University Press, 1991: 279-297.
74. Jerne NK, Henry C, Nordin AA, Fuji H, Koros AMC, Lefkovits I. Plaque-forming cells: Methodology and theory. Transpl Rev 1974; 18:130-191.
75. Lorenzen J, Lewis CE, McCracken D, Horak E, Greenall M, McGee JO'D. Human tumor-associated NK cells secrete increased amounts of interferon-γ and interleukin-4. Br J Cancer 1991; 64:457-462.
76. Lewis CE, McCracken D, Ling R, Richards PS, McCarthy SP, McGee JO'D. Cytokine release by single, immunophenotyped human cells: Use of the reverse hemolytic plaque assay. Immunol Rev 1991; 119:23-39.
77. Rabinowich H, Vitolo D, Altarac S, Herberman RB, Whiteside TL. Role of cytokines in the adoptive immunotherapy of an experimental model of human head and neck cancer by human IL-2-activated natural killer cells. J Immunol 1992; 149:340-349.

CHAPTER 3

METHODS FOR ISOLATION OF TIL FROM HUMAN SOLID TUMORS

The ability to obtain TIL and tumor cells with consistently high yield and viability from human tumor biopsy specimens is essential for studies of TIL and for cellular AIT with TIL. Viable tumor cells are required for the in vitro analysis of antitumor function of TIL and for in vitro-sensitization (IVS) protocols, when attempts are made to culture cytolytic T cells from TIL. Generally, the recovery of viable cells from tumor depends on its type and size, degree of cellular infiltration, extent of tumor necrosis, and expertise of a laboratory in tumor processing.

Procedures for disaggregation of human solid tumors that maximize tumor cell or TIL yield and viability without altering tumor cell immunogenicity or TIL growth potential have been recently developed.[1-3] Mechanical or enzymatic methods alone or in combination have been most commonly used in preparation of single cell suspensions from human solid tumors. The method of choice for TIL separation is often dependent upon the particular tumor type or requirements of a clinical treatment protocol. For many tumors, mechanical disaggregation alone is either ineffective or too damaging to tumor cells. Likewise, low viability and poor recovery of TIL are often associated with the use of mechanical methods. Most solid tumors can be effectively processed using a combination of mild mechanical and enzymatic disaggregation. After single cell suspensions are obtained, the separation of tumor cells from TIL can be accomplished by discontinuous density gradient centrifugation on, e.g., preformed differential Ficoll-Hypaque gradients or Percoll gradients.[2,4] A routine method for processing of human solid tumors which is applicable to a wide range of tumor types and clinical protocols and which has been used in our own laboratory with considerable success is described.[1-3]

TISSUE COLLECTION AND PROCESSING

Tumor tissues are collected during surgery and, thereafter, handled under sterile conditions. Tissues placed in sterile containers or bags are immediately hand-carried to the hospital Surgical Pathology Laboratory. Timing is important, because of autolysis that might be occurring in tissue, and no more than one to two hours should pass between surgery and tissue processing. It is always best to have a pathologist sample the tumor tissue in the operating room (OR). For this procedure to work, sterile gloves, forceps, scalpels and containers with media (Hanks balanced salt solution [HBSS] or

RPMI) must be available at all times in the OR (can be prepared ahead of time) to be used by the pathologist for sampling of tumor tissue. As large a sample of viable tumor as possible should be reserved for processing after the tissue required for the pathologic diagnosis has been taken. Once sampled, the tissue should be transported to the laboratory in a container of cold transport medium. Sterile physiologic saline can be substituted, provided the sample is handled quickly. It is essential that the tissue should not dry out. The container containing the tumor tissue should be labeled with the patient's name, identification number, and date as well as time of surgery.

The tumor tissue is processed using sterile techniques in a laminar flow hood. First, the tissue specimen is trimmed of fat, connective tissue, and obvious necrotic areas and weighed. The wet weight of the tumor is recorded. Next, the tumor is minced with scalpels to obtain pieces no larger than 5 mm in diameter. The minced tissue fragments are washed in HBSS to remove cellular debris and red blood cells. This can be accomplished by gravity sedimentation or by using a Cellector with a 50 or 100 mesh screen. The clean fragments are then enzymatically digested in a trypsinizing flask on a submersible magnetic stirrer in a 37°C water bath. A sufficient volume of enzyme cocktail (collagenase, DNAse and hyaluronidase) is added to completely cover the tissue fragments.[3] Care must be taken to employ a minimal rate of stirring so that tissue is not damaged. The digestion can be done at room temperature and without stirring, but the amount of time required for complete digestion will be increased. Digestion proceeds for 30–45 minutes and is repeated as required (sometimes three to four times, if the tumor is large) with fresh enzyme cocktail until all tissue fragments are digested. The concentration of collagenase, DNAse, and hyaluronidase may be increased or decreased depending upon the tissue to be digested. In general, the more connective tissue in the specimen, the higher the enzyme concentrations employed to optimize the digestion process. The digest is filtered through sterile 50–90 μ nylon mesh to separate large cell aggregates and undigested tissue from small aggregates and single cells. The pore size of the nylon mesh used will vary depending on the size of the tumor cells and whether or not aggregates are to be excluded in the final cell preparation. The filtered digest is centrifuged promptly at 250 x g for ten minutes and cells resuspended in wash medium (RPMI). Centrifugation is repeated to wash out enzymes from the cell preparation. Next, cells are examined microscopically for viability (trypan blue dye exclusion) and the presence of tumor and TIL. When enzymatic digestion is complete, all of the washed cell suspensions are pooled together and cells counted on a hema–cytometer in trypan blue dye. The number and viability of recovered tumor cells and TIL are recorded.

The tissue processing methods described above may have to be varied, depending on tumor type or size. Also, modifications of this generalized procedure may be necessary, depending on the intended use of the recovered cells.

BANKING OF TIL AND TUMOR CELLS

Depending on the ultimate use of the cells, it may be necessary to cryopreserve tumor and/or TIL. This can be done using rate-controlled freezing in a Cryomed at a rate of -1°C per minute to -40°C and then quickly to -90°C. The cells are resuspended in human AB serum in one-half the final volume and twice the final cell concentration ($5–10 \times 10^6$) required for cryopreservation. The cells are kept on ice and an equal volume of cold 2x freeze medium (RPMI containing human serum and dimethyl sulfoxide, DMSO) is slowly added drop by drop to the cell suspension.[3] One milliliter of this cell suspension is added to freezing vials, which are immediately placed in the rate-controlled freezer. Vials are stored in vapor phase in a liquid nitrogen storage unit. The method used for thawing cells is as important as that for cryopreservation for recovery of viable cells. Cells are quickly thawed in a 37°C water bath and then diluted slowly (drop by drop) with warm medium containing 5% (v/v) serum. The recovered cells are washed twice to remove residual DMSO and their viability and cell number determined to calculate recovery. Cryopreserved tumor cells and TIL can be successfully used for a variety of studies and for expansion in culture. For therapeutic culture of TIL, it is preferable to utilize freshly separated rather than banked TIL (Chapter 8).

GRADIENTS FOR SEPARATION OF TIL AND TUMOR CELLS

Separation of TIL from human tumor biopsies presents a unique problem in that often only small biopsy specimens are available. Among 40 consecutive tumor biopsies in our institution, an average weight of specimens was about 3 g wet weight. The number of viable cells in disaggregated tumor tissue varied but was seldom larger than 10 x 10^7 cells and often smaller. For separation of TIL from tumor cells in human tumors, it is essential to have a method that is rapid, easy and adaptable to relatively small numbers of cells recovered from surgical biopsies. The method of choice should achieve satisfactory separation, yield cells that are viable and functionally intact, give good recovery and avoid selective losses of cell populations.

A variety of cell separation methods have been used for TIL.[4] Of the two methods most commonly employed, velocity sedimentation is based primarily on cell size, while gradient centrifugation depends on differences in density as well as size between the cells in suspension. In earlier studies, discontinuous density gradients have been successfully used by Vose et al,[5] Vose[6] and Klein et al[7] for separations of infiltrating leukocytes and tumor cells[8] from a variety of human tumors. Other investigators used one-step isopycnic density gradients[9] or discontinuous Percoll gradients[10] for purification of tumor cells. Pretlow and Pretlow[4] explicitly stated that density gradients are unsatisfactory for separations of cell mixtures in which densities of different cell types are likely to overlap. Nevertheless, we resorted to these gradients as an easy, time-saving alternative to velocity sedimentation at unit gravity.[1,2] Our comparisons of the two methods indicated that

Table 1. Cellular composition of the TIL-enriched fractions isolated from six human melanomas and separated on different gradients[a]

	Velocity sedimentation gradient n=3	Density gradient n=3
Lymphocytes	45 ± 15 (34 - 56)	43 ± 2 (40 - 44)
Monocytes/macrophages	2 ± 0.4 (0 - 4)	1 ± 1.7 (0 - 3)
Granulocytes	4 ± 1 (3 - 5)	2 ± 1.5 (0 - 3)
Nonhematopoietic cells[b]	50 ± 12 (42 - 58)	50 ± 9 (40 - 56)

[a] Determined by morphology on Wright/Giemsa or May-Grunwald-Giemsa (MGG) smears. 150-200 cells/smear were counted. Data presented as mean percentages ± SD. Ranges are given in parentheses.
[b] Tumor cells, tissue cells and cells that could not be identified.
(From Whiteside et al, J Immunol Methods 1986;90:221-233)

there was little difference in the cellular composition of TIL-enriched fractions recovered. The enrichment in TIL was also comparable (about 30–40 fold) and the viability of recovered TIL was always >95%.

In our experience, using either velocity sedimentation or discontinuous density gradients adapted to small volumes and relatively low numbers of cells, satisfactory preparations enriched in TIL can be obtained from human solid tumors. The two methods are comparable in terms of recovery, purity and cellular composition of the TIL fractions. However, density gradients were found to be simpler, less time-consuming and more practical for routine preparations of TIL from clinical material than velocity sedimentation.[1,2] As shown in Table 1, cellular composition of the TIL-enriched fractions separated either by velocity sedimentation or discontinuous density gradients from enzymatic digests of human melanomas was almost identical.[2] Note that nonhematopoietic (largely tumor) cells represented a considerable component of the TIL fractions shown in Table 1. In contrast, with enzymatic digests of some breast carcinomas, separation on discontinuous density gradients resulted in a high degree of purity of both TIL and tumor cell fractions (Fig. 1). In tumors that gave highly-enriched TIL and tumor fractions, a substantial loss of cells was invariably observed, and the recovery could be as low as 5–10%. Thus, it is not unusual with discontinuous or differential density gradients to achieve excellent separation of TIL with poor recovery or, conversely, poor separation of TIL from tumor cells with recovery of 50–90%. As individual tumors are heterogeneous in terms of both cell size and cell density,[2] it is difficult to predict their behavior during a separation procedure.

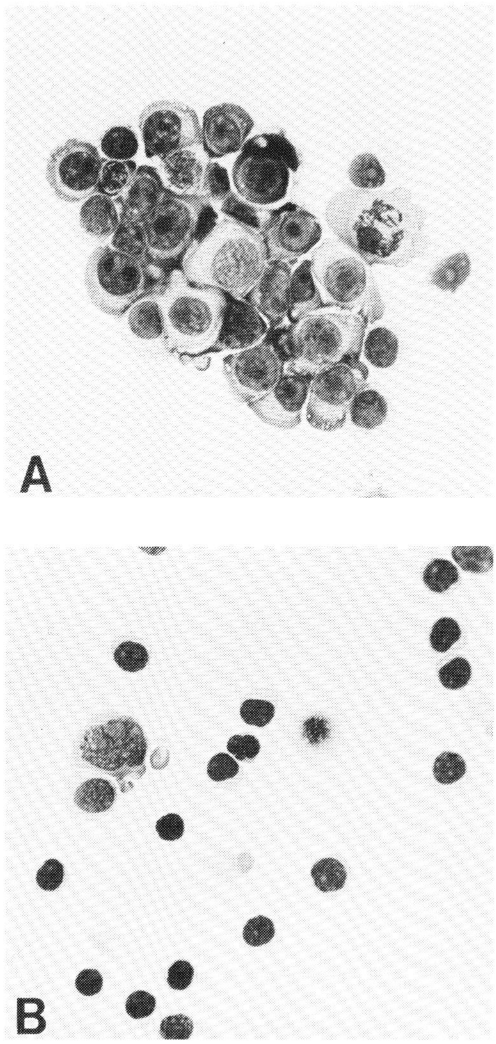

Fig. 1. Tumor cell fraction in a and TIL-enriched fraction in b obtained by centrifugation of an enzymatic digest of human breast carcinoma on a discontinuous density gradient. May-Grünwald-Giemsa stain. Mag x 1000. Reproduced with permission from Whiteside et al, J Immunol Methods 1986;90:221-233.

CRITERIA FOR EVALUATING TIL PURITY AND RECOVERY

After TIL and tumor cells are isolated and separated, their purity and recovery need to be determined and recorded. The recovery is usually expressed as the number of cells recovered per gram of wet weight of tumor tissue. However, although widely used, this estimate of recovery is not informative: a gram of tumor tissue yields variable numbers of cells depending on the tumor size, location, degree of infiltration with inflammatory cells, completeness of disaggregation, and skills of a technologist in minimizing the cell loss. But mainly, the formula for calculating recovery of cells from tumors does not indicate the real number of starting cells, which is essential for monitoring the process of recovery. It is perhaps best to determine the number of MNC and tumor cells in the final tumor digest by performing a viable cell count with a trypan blue dye and, using these estimates as a starting point, to express recovery as the number of recovered TIL or tumor cells relative to the starting number in the suspension per gram of tissue. The viability of recovered cells should be >95%, particularly since they are often destined to be cryopreserved. In general, both the viability and recovery of TIL are much better than those of tumor cells, which tend to die, clump or sediment during the process of recovery on density gradients. Recoveries of TIL from human tumor biopsies cannot be predicted on the basis of tumor or biopsy size, but they may reflect the degree of tumor infiltration with MNC. For example, recovery of TIL from a small series of 13 breast tumors in our hands varied from 6×10^3 to 7×10^6 per gram of wet tumor tissue.[11] In this study, the number of T lymphocytes recovered from tumors was compared to that counted in immunoperoxidase-stained sections. While there was no relationship between in situ counts and the T-cell recovery in individual cases, as a group, tumors which were densely infiltrated in situ tended to yield more T lymphocytes per gram tumor weight than tumors with scarce infiltrates.[11] To give another example of TIL recovery, from 70 liver tumors (26 primary; 40 metastatic-mostly from the colon; 4 benign) studied in our laboratory, we recovered on the average $0.8 \pm 0.2 \times 10^6$ TIL/g (mean ± SD), with a range of $0–9.2 \times 10^6$ TIL/g.

The purity of recovered enriched TIL or tumor cell fractions is estimated morphologically on cytocentrifuge smears stained with May-Grunwald-Giemsa (MGG). It varies widely for different tumors processed in the same way. In the example of 13 breast tumors given above, the TIL enriched fraction was found to contain 66.4% ± 22 of lymphocytes (means ± SD); 2% ± 2 of monocytes/macrophages; 1.2% ± 1 granulocytes; rare basophils, and 30% ± 23 of tumor and other nonhematopoietic cells.[11] The purity greater than 70% is difficult to achieve for TIL and usually requires more than one gradient separation or an additional enrichment step, such as panning on antibody-coated plates or complement-dependent lysis. Of course, when good purity of TIL is desired, the recovery is likely to be compromised. An investigator needs to decide at the start whether to aim for purity of TIL or for their maximal recovery. It is necessary to bear in mind that highly enriched TIL preparations may not be representative, as cell losses occurring during purification may not only be substantial but also selective.

Table 2. Tumor-infiltrating lymphocytes (TIL) from human solid tumors: Number of T lymphocytes recovered from TIL suspensions following separation by sorting[a]

Tumors	Biopsy weight (g)	% $CD2^+$ in initial TIL suspensions	No. of $CD2^+$ cells recovered by sorting
n = 15	3.4 (0.2 - 29)	26 (11 - 69)	3×10^5 (6×10^4 - 1×10^6)

[a] TIL recovered from 14 different solid tumors (carcinomas of the ovary, breast, lung, colon, esophagus) and one ascites fluid were enriched by centrifugation on differential Ficoll-Hypaque gradients, stained with anti-CD2 mAb, and sorted by flow cytometry. The recovered viable $CD2^+$ cells were counted with the aid of trypan blue. The data are presented as medians, with ranges in parentheses. The data were obtained by Dr. Sylvia Miescher, Ludwig Institute for Cancer Research, Lausanne, Switzerland.

(From Whiteside in Lotzova E, Herberman RB, eds. Interleukin 2 and Killer Cells in Cancer, CRC Press 1990; pp. 133-151)

Highly purified fresh TIL can also be obtained by sorting of partially-enriched cell suspensions on a flow cytometer. The numbers of highly purified, FACS-sorted TIL-T lymphocytes are often limited. However. Table 2 summarizes the recoveries of $CD2^+$ TIL-T, following sorting of cell suspensions obtained from 15 solid tumors of different histologic types. The small numbers of recovered TIL-T preclude extensive functional analysis, but they are, nevertheless, sufficient for a partial characterization of these cells in different TIL preparations. Using FACS-purified T lymphocytes, we showed that T cells isolated from human solid tumors expressed the CD3-Ti complex on their membranes, as determined by reactivity with anti-CD3 and WT31 mAbs.[12] The expression of the β chains of the TcR was comparable on the surface of TIL-T and normal PBL-T.[12]

SUMMARY

The procedure for TIL isolation from surgical tumor biopsies has been recently optimized, based on extensive experience of many investigators with various types of tumors in the last ten years. The isolation process, consisting of a combination of mild enzymatic digestion and gentle mechanical disaggregation, facilitates separation of TIL from tumor cells, attempts to decrease selective losses of cellular populations and to increase recovery of cells with good purity and viability. The wider application of standardized methods for TIL recovery from solid tumor tissue is likely to diminish differences in phenotypic and functional characteristics of TIL between different laboratories. However, even the most precise and well-controlled processing will not substitute for the quality of tumor biopsy: fresh and carefully sampled tumor specimens in respect to size, location of the sample in the tumor (i.e., samples from tumor border are often better infiltrated than the center of tumor) or a degree of tumor necrosis (very large tumors tend to be necrotic), are essential for successful TIL recovery. For tumors that are surgically removed with an intent to use TIL for AIT, special handling is necessary to assure that tissue is placed in sterile medium immediately after excision and processed for TIL recovery as soon as possible.

REFERENCES

1. Whiteside TL, Miescher S, Hurlimann J, Von Fliedner V. Separation, phenotyping and limiting-dilution analysis of T lymphocytes infiltrating human solid tumors. Int J Cancer 1986; 37:803-811.
2. Whiteside TL, Miescher S, MacDonald RH, Von Fliedner V. Separation of tumor-infiltrating lymphocytes from tumor cells in human solid tumors. A comparison between velocity sedimentation and discontinuous density gradients. J Immunol Methods 1986; 90:221-233.
3. Elder E, Whiteside TL. Processing of tumors for vaccine and/or tumor-infiltrating lymphocytes. In: Rose N, DeMacario EC, Fahey JL, Friedman H, Penn GM., eds. Manual of Clinical Laboratory Immunology. Washington,DC: ASM, 1993: 817-819.
4. Pretlow TP, Pretlow TG. Cell Separation: Methods and Selected Applications. New York:Academic Press, 1986.
5. Vose BM, Vanky F, Klein E. Lymphocyte cytotoxicity against autologous tumor biopsy cells in humans. Int J Cancer 1977; 20:512-519.
6. Vose BM. Separation of tumor and host cell populations from human neoplasms. In: Reid E., ed.Methodologic surveys. Chichester: Ellis Harwood, 1982: 45-56.
7. Klein E, Vanky F, Galili V, Vose B, Fopp M. Separation and characteristics of tumor-infiltrating lymphocytes in man. In: Witz IP, Hanna Jr, MG, eds.Contemporary Topics in Immunology. New York: Plenum Press, 1980: 79-107.
8. Yanagawa E, Uchida A, Moore M, Micksche M. Autologous tumor killing and natural cytotoxic activity of tumor-associated macrophages in cancer patients. Cancer Immunol Immunother 1985; 19:163-167.
9. Stackpole CW, Cremona P, Kassel RL. Metrizamide gradient purification of mouse tumor cells. J Immunol 1979; 30:231-243.
10. Kedar E, Ikejiri BL, Bonnard GD, Herberman RB. A rapid technique for isolation of viable tumor cells from solid tumors: Use of the tumor cells for induction

and measurement of cell-mediated cytotoxic responses. Eur J Cancer Clin Oncol 1982; 18:991-1000.

11. Whiteside TL, Miescher S, Hurlimann J, Moretta L, Von Fliedner V. Clonal analysis and in situ characterization of lymphocytes infiltrating human breast carcinomas. Cancer Immunol Immunother 1986; 23:169-178.

12. Miescher S, Stoeck M, Qiao L, Barras C, Barrelet L, Von Fliedner V. Proliferative and cytolytic potentials of purified human tumor-infiltrating T lymphocytes. Impaired response to mitogen-driven stimulation despite T-cell receptor expression. Int J Cancer 1988; 42:659-666.

CHAPTER 4

Morphologic and Phenotypic Characteristics of Freshly Isolated TIL

TIL isolated from surgically removed tumor specimens by enzymatic digestion and density gradient centrifugation, as described in Chapter 3, represent mixtures of T lymphocytes and tumor cells with different proportions of macrophages, granulocytes, eosinophils and large granular lymphocytes (LGL). In order to isolate TIL for phenotypic or functional analyses, further purification steps are generally necessary. These can be accomplished by a variety of well-established methods, from sorting by flow cytometry, additional gradient separations, positive or negative selection with mAbs, to rosetting with sheep erythrocytes.[1] Due to the small number of TIL generally recovered, these purification procedures might have to be scaled down. Morphologic examination of TIL on stained cytocentrifuge smears is both easy and informative in regard to cell types present in TIL preparations. Phenotypic analyses of TIL by flow cytometry can be performed on suspensions of enzymatically-disaggregated biopsies, but might encounter difficulties in gating if there is a substantial contamination with tumor cells or their fragments. Phenotypic analyses of TIL by immunohistology on cytocentrifuge smears are possible and have been used to monitor fresh TIL preparations. During TIL purification, it might be preferable to avoid too many additional steps for fear of selective losses of TIL subpopulations. Finally, although TIL isolated as described in Chapter 3 are mainly T lymphocytes, it is necessary to remember that macrophages are the other prominent MNC in tumors, and that a different isolation procedure would be needed if phenotypic characterization of tumor-associated macrophages (TAM) is desired.

MORPHOLOGY OF ISOLATED TIL

On MGG-stained smears of enzymatic digests of tumor tissues, TIL have morphologic characteristics of small lymphocytes (Fig. 1a). A small proportion of TIL in these preparations may look like LGL (Fig. 1b). Following centrifugation on a differential gradient to remove tumor cells, morphology of TIL closely resembles that of PBL. The average size of TIL is 10 μm.[2] This appears to be in conflict with the immunohistologic data reviewed in Chapter 2 and with flow cytometry results discussed below, which indicate that a considerable proportion of TIL expresses activation

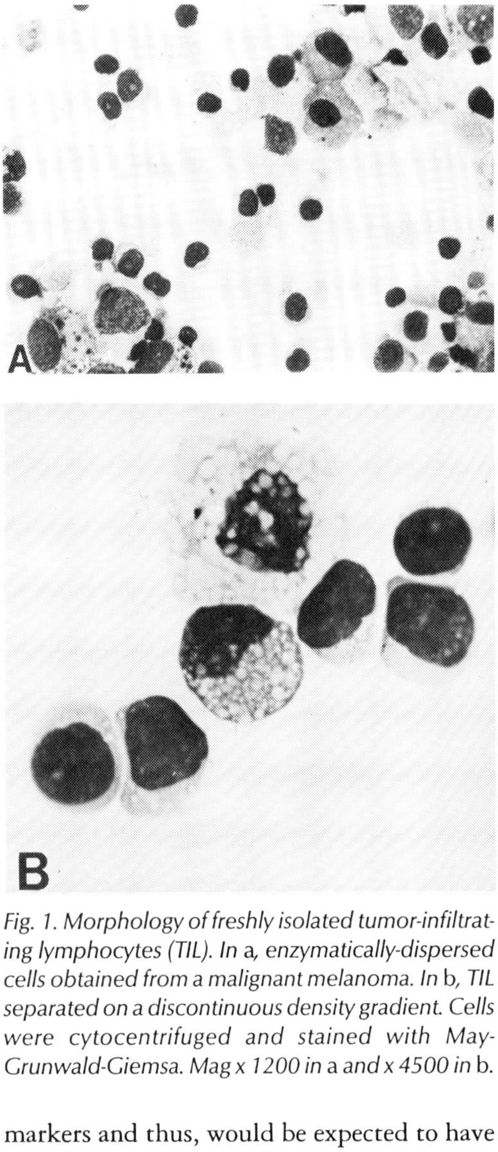

Fig. 1. Morphology of freshly isolated tumor-infiltrating lymphocytes (TIL). In a, enzymatically-dispersed cells obtained from a malignant melanoma. In b, TIL separated on a discontinuous density gradient. Cells were cytocentrifuged and stained with May-Grunwald-Giemsa. Mag x 1200 in a and x 4500 in b.

markers and thus, would be expected to have morphology of activated lymphocytes, which are larger, have a higher cytoplasm/nucleus ratio, and contain more cytoplasmic granules than resting lymphocytes. It has been suggested that activated lymphocytes have a tendency to adhere to tumor cells forming conjugates, which are either pelleted during centrifugation or are present, in part, in the tumor cell fraction. Such conjugates have been observed in enzymatic digests of tumor tissue.[3] However, examination of tumor cells separated on differential gradients have not confirmed the presence of lymphocyte tumor cell conjugates in any substantial proportions. Also, by flow cytometry, some TIL in a lymphogate consistently express activation Ags. This implies that activated, and perhaps functionally most relevant cells, have not been lost during the process of purification. The presence of activation markers on morphologically small lymphocytes suggests that TIL might be arrested early in the activation process and have failed to proceed to the blast form in the tumor microenvironment. This hypothesis is supported by functional studies of TIL, as described in Chapter 5.

TWO-COLOR FLOW CYTOMETRY ANALYSIS OF TIL

Two-color flow cytometry has been extensively used for the phenotypic analysis of fresh TIL suspensions. In contrast to immunohistology, which utilizes fresh-frozen or fixed tumor tissues, flow cytometry is generally performed on freshly-isolated TIL. In this way, chances of denaturation of more sensitive surface Ags on TIL are eliminated as is a bias, which is always associated with visual enumeration of lymphocytes in tissue by eye. Flow cytometry results are objective and also more reliable, as at least 5,000 events are generally recorded. The amount of fluorochrome on each cell, as shown by the brightness of the signal, reflects the amount of cell surface marker allowing semi-quantification. The use of two fluorochromes simultaneously makes possible the analysis of two coincident surface markers, e.g., a phenotypic marker and an activation marker. The use of propidium iodide to stain the dead cells allows their exclusion from the analysis and, therefore, eliminates nonspecific binding to cytoplasmic proteins.

The availability of mAbs specific for adhesion molecules, activation Ags, cytokine receptors and the TcR Ags has allowed for further phenotypic characterization of TIL by flow cytometry. The number of recovered TIL is often a limiting factor, however, and the relevant phenotypic data cannot always be determined, particularly when functional studies are a priority.

Flow cytometry of fresh TIL preparations facilitates utilization of a broader array and different combinations of mAbs than immunohistology, allowing for a more complete discrimination between different subpopulations of lymphoid cells. In our laboratory, the phenotypic characteristics of TIL obtained from several types of human tumors (melanoma, breast, ovarian or colon carcinoma, SCCHN, hepatocellular carcinoma) have been compared to those observed by immunohistology and found to be similar. Three points are worth emphasizing: (a) among CD3$^+$ cells, which are the major cellular component of TIL, up to 25% and 65% express CD25 and HLA-DR Ags (activation markers), respectively, in some tumor types (e.g., ovarian carcinomas, see Fig. 2); (b) some TIL preparations may contain variable and sometimes considerable proportions of CD3$^-$CD56$^+$ NK cells and CD3$^+$CD56$^+$ non-MHC-restricted T lymphocytes; and (c) the CD4/CD8 ratios are variable but often are greater than one, indicating that in many tumors, CD4$^+$ rather than CD8$^+$ T lymphocytes predominate.

THE CD4/CD8 RATIO IN TIL

Several recent studies have indicated that the CD4/CD8 ratio in fresh TIL isolated from metastatic melanomas,[4] RCC,[5] and primary breast[6] and lung cancer[7] may be significantly reduced as a result of enrichment in CD8$^+$ cells. In contrast, in nonmalignant inflammatory exudates the majority of T cells have been observed to express the CD4$^+$ phenotype.[8,9] It has also been suggested that the content of CD8$^+$ T lymphocytes in at least some human solid tumors may have prognostic significance.[10,11] However, evidence for prognostic significance of CD8$^+$ infiltrates in the tumor is not consistent. We have addressed this issue in one small study using TIL from patients with SCCHN.[12] The study was performed with TIL from 17 SCCHN patients, and it showed that the low TIL CD4/CD8 ratio in 8 patients at the time of surgery, due in part to a significant ($p<0.001$) increase in CD8$^+$ and in part to a decrease in CD4$^+$ cells ($p<0.01$) was associated with the absence of extracapsular spread and cervical metastases (Table 1) and thus a better prognosis.[12] On the other hand, the high CD4/CD8 ratio seen in the other 9 patients could be related to extracapsular spread in 86% and cervical lymph node metastases in 78% of patients at the time of surgery and thus to a poor prognosis.[12] Further analysis of a relationship between the TIL characteristics and tumor recurrence and survival of the patients is needed to confirm these

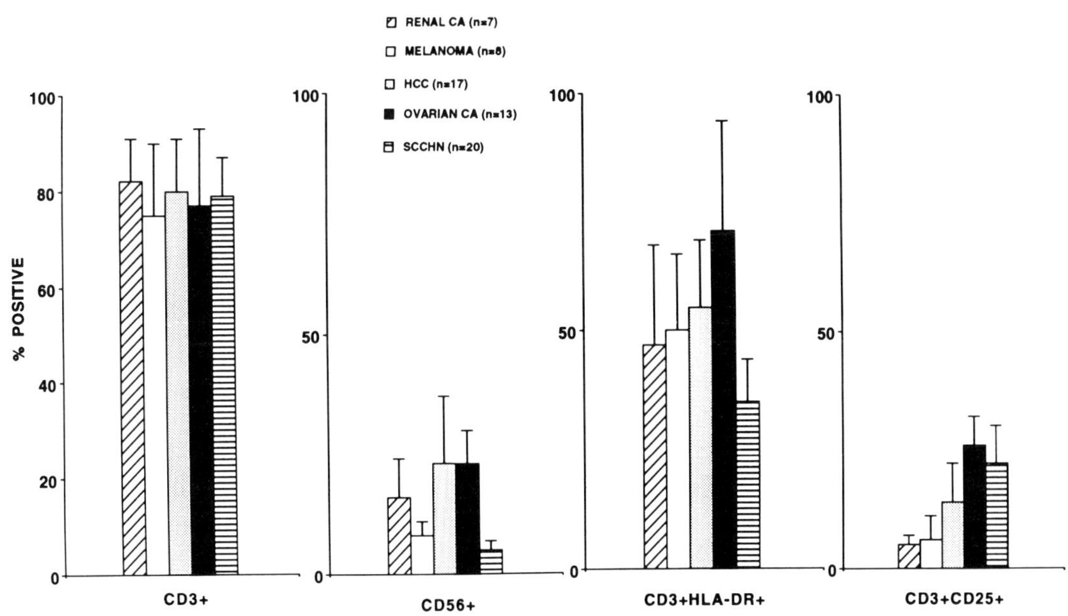

Fig. 2. Phenotypic characteristics of tumor-infiltrating lymphocytes freshly isolated from various human tumors by density centrifugation and stained with mAbs for two-color flow cytometry.

Table 1. The CD4/CD8 ratio and prognostic factors in two groups of fresh TIL obtained from tumor biopsies of patients with squamous cell carcinoma of the head and neck

	n = 8	n = 9	
CD4/CD8	0.5 ± 0.3	2.6 ± 1.7	p<0.005
% CD4$^+$	23 ± 12	40 ± 13	p<0.01
% CD8$^+$	44 ± 8	19 ± 10	p<0.001
Cervical mets[a]	2/8 (25%)	7/9 (78%)	p<0.004
ECS[a]	None	6/7 (86%)	p<0.001

[a] ECS (extracapsular spread) and cervical metastases were evaluated at the time of surgery. TIL were isolated from surgical tumor biopsies and phenotyped as described in Table 2. The patients were divided into two groups on the basis of the CD4/CD8 ratios observed in TIL suspensions. Data are presented as means ± SD. Differences between the two groups were calculated by Student's t-test.

observations. Still, our study and those of others suggest that the composition of the host's TIL may have prognostic importance in at least some human tumors.[10,13]

Flow cytometry analysis of TIL and A-PBL have been performed to determine whether phenotypic differences can be found between these cell populations. As shown in Table 2, which summarizes data from our laboratory for human SCCHN, CD3$^+$ T lymphocytes were the major TIL subpopulation.[12,14] The TIL contained significantly fewer NK cells than A-PBL. The proportion of activated T cells was significantly (<0.05) increased in TIL suspensions. The latter had a reduced CD4/CD8 cell ratio, and this was due mainly to the lower proportion of CD4$^+$ cells in TIL, as compared to A-PBL.[12,13,15] As a result of this type of comparisons, it has been possible to confirm that TIL freshly-isolated from several different types of human tumors are phenotypically distinct from A-PBL,[15] being often enriched in CD8$^+$ T cells.

Using flow cytometry, the cellular phenotype of TIL recovered from primary versus metastatic human tumors was also compared in our laboratory, using flow cytometry. As shown in Table 3, there were no significant differences detected between the fresh TIL populations obtained from primary or metastatic liver tumors.[16] The mean CD4/CD8 ratios for TIL from primary and metastatic liver tumors were 1.3 and 1.1, respectively.

Table 2. Phenotypic analysis of fresh TIL and A-PBL from patients with squamous cell carcinomas of the head and neck[a]

Phenotype	TIL (n = 17)	A-PBL (n = 17)
	% positive	
CD3$^+$	80 ± 9	70 ± 11
CD2$^+$	84 ± 8	78 ± 18
CD4$^+$	33 ± 13	44 ± 17
CD8$^+$	32 ± 16	30 ± 15
Leu19$^+$	3 ± 2*	10 ± 2
CD16$^+$	4 ± 3*	21 ± 26
CD4/CD8	1	1.5
CD3$^+$Leu19$^+$	2 ± 1.7	5 ± 5
CD3$^+$IL-2R$^+$	14 ± 11*	7 ± 6
CD2$^+$HLA-DR$^+$	29 ± 17*	5 ± 4
CD16$^+$/CD8$^+$	1 ± 1	4 ± 4

[a] Data are presented as means ± SD. All tumors were primary and the TIL were recovered from fresh tumor biopsies as described in the text. TIL or A-PBL were incubated with labeled mAbs to lymphocyte surface antigens washed in PBS-Na azide buffer, and analyzed by two-color flow cytometry in a FACStar instrument. Asterisks indicate significant differences (p<0.05) between TIL and A-PBL.

(From Whiteside in Lotzova E, Herberman RB, eds. Interleukin 2 and Killer Cells in Cancer, CRC Press 1990:pp. 133-151)

Table 3. Phenotypic analysis of freshly isolated tumor-infiltrating lymphocytes (TIL) and peripheral blood lymphocytes (PBL) from human liver tumors[a]

	TIL (%)		PBL (%) (n=6)
	Primary (n=5)	Metastatic (n=5)	
$CD3^+$	71 ± 6	79 ± 2	64 ± 2
$CD4^+$	39 ± 3	38 ± 8	37 ± 7
$CD8^+$	29 ± 2	34 ± 10	30 ± 4
$CD56^+(NKH1^+)$	25 ± 4[b]	21 ± 3[b]	12 ± 2
$CD3^+CD56^+$	14 ± 4	11 ± 3	6 ± 2
$CD25^+$	11 ± 3[b]	16 ± 4[b]	4 ± 1
$CD3^+CD25^+$	10 ± 1[b]	14 ± 1[b]	3 ± 1
$HLA\text{-}DR^+$	55 ± 5[b]	55 ± 5[b]	20 ± 3
$CD3^+HLA\text{-}DR^+$	40 ± 4[b]	39 ± 3[b]	7 ± 1

[a] Lymphocytes in suspension were stained with labeled mAbs and analyzed by two-color flow cytometry. Data are presented as means ± SE.
[b] Statistically significant differences between TIL and PBL (p<0.05)

Fresh TIL contained more $CD3^+CD56^+$ T cells ($p<0.05$) than A-PBL. Also, significantly more activated ($CD3^+CD25^+$ and $CD3^+HLA\text{-}DR^+$) T cells ($p<0.01$) were present in TIL than A-PBL, indicating in situ activation of TIL or accumulation of activated T cells in both types of liver tumors.

THE PRESENCE OF ACTIVATED T CELLS IN TIL

In a recent flow cytometry study of TIL obtained from 31 patients with breast cancer, the phenotype and activation status of TIL were analyzed.[17] As usual, in all patients the predominant cells were T lymphocytes, and in the majority of cases $CD8^+$ lymphocytes were present in a greater number than $CD4^+$ lymphocytes. There was no relationship between the degree of lymphocytic infiltration and either tumor stage or grade, but there appeared to be an inverse correlation with the levels of ER in the tumor ($p<0.01$). Both populations of T cells had significantly higher numbers of cells carrying HLA-DR (class II MHC Ag) than the equivalent populations in peripheral blood from the same patient group ($p<0.001$). The transferrin receptor (CD71) was found on similar numbers of $CD8^+$ T cells in PBL and TIL, while more of the $CD4^+$ T cells infiltrating the tumor were found to carry this receptor ($p=0.034$). The IL-2R-α (CD25, Tac) Ag was also expressed on similar numbers of $CD8^+$ T cells obtained from both peripheral blood and the tumor but was present on fewer $CD4^+$ T cells in TIL as compared to PBL ($p=0.029$). In both TILs and blood lymphocytes, the IL-2R-α was consistently expressed on a greater number of $CD4^+$ than $CD8^+$ T lymphocytes ($p<0.001$). TIL obtained from human tumors were found to express IL-2R-β in the same or greater proportion of cells than A-PBL.[18,19] For example, Alexander et al found no significant difference in the percentage of $CD3^+IL\text{-}2R\text{-}\beta^+$ or the density of expression per cell in TIL versus A-PBL.[31]

NAIVE VERSUS MEMORY T CELLS IN TIL

Lymphocyte differentiation from the naive to Ag-primed or -activated state is generally accompanied by a change in the CD45 gene product on their surface. Two mutually exclusive surface markers, the CD45 Ag (leukocyte common Ag (LCA) family) on naive T cells and the CD29 Ag (β-chain of the VLA/integrin family, which includes receptors for fibronectin and other extracellular matrix molecules) on memory T cells were thought to distinguish these two subsets of $CD3^+$ lymphocytes.[20] The CD45 Ag is a glycoprotein with a large constant cytoplasmic domain with tyrosine phosphatase activity,[21] a short transmembrane domain and an extracellular domain which can be expressed in several isoforms due to alternative splicing of the exons A,B,C[22] and differential glycosylation,[23] resulting in molecular weights varying from 180-220 kD. Naive T cells are characterized by the expression of the highest molecular weight form of the CD45 Ag (now named CD45RA, detected by the mAbs 2H4,[24] HB-aa, SN130, and Leu18) and a lack of expression of the lowest molecular weight form (named CD45RO), detected by the mAb UCHL-1[25]) as well as a lack of CD29 (detected by the mAb 4B4[26]). In addition, the CD45RA Ag disappears from the surface after Ag exposure of immature or naive T-cells, whereas the CD45RO and CD29 Ags become increasingly and permanently expressed, thus qualifying as permanent activation markers.[27-29] But it has recently become clear that naive T cells do not completely lack CD45RO and CD29 Ag, nor do they lose the CD45RA isoform completely after antigenic or mitogenic stimulation in vitro, and the terms "positive/negative" were replaced by "high/low" expression.[20]

In our own studies and those of others, the majority of TIL has been consistently found to express CD29 Ags.[30] However, considerable variability in the ratio of memory to naive T cells existed between different tumors, although this ratio was almost always greater among $CD4^+$ than $CD8^+$ TIL (see Fig. 3).[18,30] This may mean that fewer $CD8^+$ than $CD4^+$ TIL-T are primed in the tumor bed. Alexander et al, analyzing TIL samples from 32 patients with RCC, showed that $CD45RA^+$ cells were significantly decreased and $CD29^+$ cells increased ($p<0.0001$ for each), with the $CD45RO^+/CD45RA^+$ ratio of 1:1 in PBL, 7:1 in $CD8^+$ TIL, and 25:1 in $CD4^+$ TIL.[31] The very high ratios of memory/naive T cells reported by Alexander et al[18,31,32] for TIL obtained from RCC may reflect true biologic differences between this and other solid tumor types or technical differences, e.g., inclusion of dimly-stained $CD45RA^+$ cells into the positive cell fraction during flow cytometry.

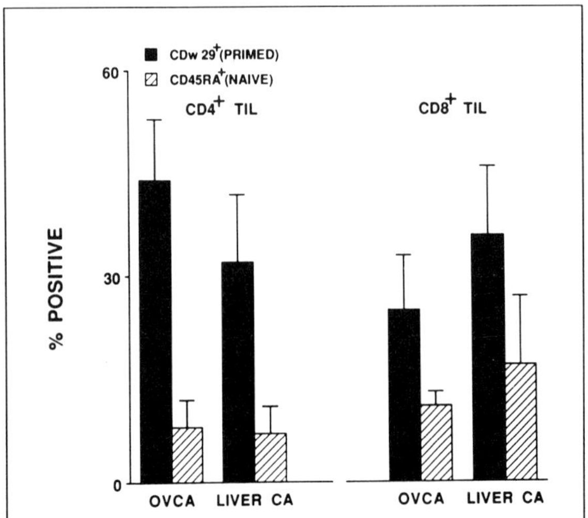

Fig. 3. Two-color flow cytometry analysis of tumor-infiltrating lymphocytes obtained from human ovarian or liver carcinomas and stained with mAbs detecting primed (anti-CDw29) or naive (anti-CD45RA) T lymphocytes.

In all situations involving participation of T cells responding to chronic antigenic stimulation, it has been documented that lymphocytes found intralesionally or perivascularly expressed CD45RO and/or CD29 Ags to a higher degree than PBL. This was true not only for tuberculoid (but not lepromatous) leprosy, *leishmania braziliensis*, rheumatoid arthritis, multiple sclerosis, atopic dermatitis, Graves disease, and tuberculous granulomas,[33-39] but also for malignant melanoma.[4] In melanoma, a significantly higher ratio between $CD29^+/CD45RA^+$ of about 7:1 for $CD4^+$ cells was found in subcutaneous metastatic deposits, although not lymph node metastases, where a "contamination" with residual original lymph node lymphocytes may interfere with the analysis.[4]

The biologic significance of the intralesional accumulation in tumors or other sites of chronic inflammation of cells with high expression of the permanent activation markers CD29/CD45RO, and low expression of the CD45RA Ag is not precisely understood. It has long been known that chronic inflammatory infiltrates are associated with local enhanced permeability of the EC layer, mainly in capillaries and in postcapillary venules.[40-42] Also, adherence of T lymphocytes to EC is the key event in the process of their extravasation into the perivascular tissue.[43] It has been shown that $CD29^+$ $CD45RO^+$ lymphocytes are more likely to interact with the EC using both type-1 (CD11a/CD18-CD54) and type-2 (CD2-CD58) intercellular adhesion pathways.[44] The resulting lymphocyte-EC contact leads to a significantly enhanced transendothelial albumin clearance, especially, if $CD29^+CD45RO^+$ lymphocytes are previously stimulated with either anti-CD3 or anti-CD28 mAb.[44] The increase in permeability perhaps induced by activated CD29+ CD45RO+ T cells could facilitate attraction and activation of additional immune cells into the tumor.

THE PRESENCE OF NK AND γ/δ T CELLS AMONG TIL

By flow cytometry, CD3-CD56+ NK cells represent a small proportion of TIL in most tumors.[30] In ovarian carcinomas, however, NK cells may be quite numerous, representing up to 25% of TIL recovered from tumor biopsies.[30,45] The paucity of NK cells in TIL obtained from tumors which are relatively advanced at the time of surgery suggests that NK cells play no major role at later stages of tumor progression. On the other hand, our observation that the proportion of NK cells is higher in LMP ovarian tumors,[46] which are often less well infiltrated than invasive ovarian carcinomas, deserves a comment. If confirmed by additional studies, this observation would suggest a role for NK cells in local antitumor responses relatively early in tumor progression. Because most human tumors contain few, if any, NK cells at the time of surgery,[47] ovarian and especially LMP tumors, might provide information about the role of NK cells in a local control of tumor growth.

In about 25% of human lung cancers, a significant proportion (10–20%) of T lymphocytes among freshly-isolated TIL was found to express the γ/δ TcR.[48,49] This interesting finding made by Zocchi and Ferrarini[48] indicated that certain human tumors may be enriched in the γ/δ+ T cells. Furthermore, these γ/δ T cells infiltrating lung adenocarcinomas selectively lysed AuTu following expansion in the presence of IL-2.[48] Similar observations were also reported from other laboratories.[49] More recently, Ferrarini et al have found that lung cancers infiltrated by γ/δ T cells expressed heat-shock protein (HSP)72 as well as the 67 kDa high-affinity laminin receptor and suggested that these tumor-associated molecules may represent Ags recognized by γ/δ+ TIL.[50] These data indicate that γ/δ+ TIL may play a role in local antitumor immunity in some cancers.

THE TCR GENE USAGE BY TIL IN SITU

It has been reported that a preferential usage of the specific TcR V β products occurs

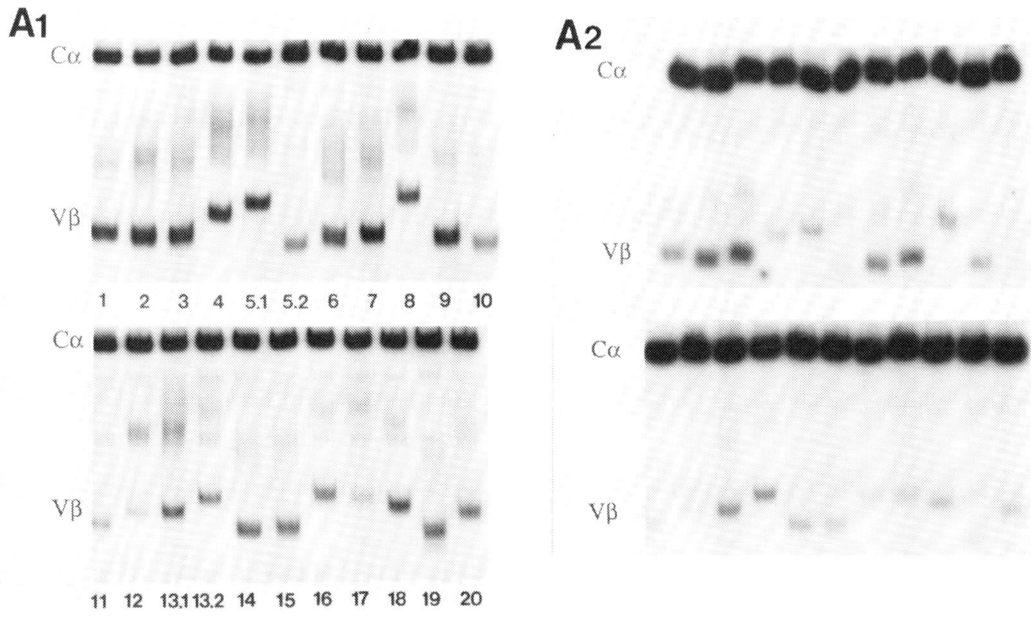

Fig. 4. T-cell receptor (TcR) V β gene expression in tumor-infiltrating lymphocytes (TIL) freshly isolated from a patient with hepatocellular carcinoma (left, A1) and from peripheral blood T cells obtained from a normal, healthy adult (right, A2). Note that while normal T cells express all the V β genes nearly equally, in TIL V β-2, V β-3 and V β-7 were more strongly expressed relative to the other V β genes. Reproduced with permission from Weidmann et al, Cancer Res 1992; 52:5913-5920.

in T cells involved in pathologic processes.[51-54] Molecular analysis of the TcR genes in TIL isolated from uveal melanoma has shown a predominant usage of the V α-7 family.[55] Studies of cultured murine or human TIL have shown preferential increases in cells expressing the TcRs of certain V β families: V β-8, V β-5, or V β-6.[56,57] The significance of the selective TcR V β usage in these cultures is still unclear and may, in fact, reflect selective proliferation in the presence of IL-2 of: (a) in vivo tumor Ag-primed T cells; (b) T cells stimulated in vitro by the AuTu; (c) preferential proliferative ability in vitro of T cells expressing certain V β genes. When TIL freshly isolated from human hepatocellular carcinomas (HCC) were studied for V β expression by quantitative PCR in our laboratory, using primers specific for different V β regions of the TcR gene, oligoclones of T cells expressing different V β genes in each tumor were identified.[58] Although the particular V β genes that were over- or underexpressed in TIL varied among the patients, in three out of five TIL the V β-3 gene was expressed with a relatively high frequency (see, e.g., Fig. 4). In contrast, the V β-4 gene was expressed with a low frequency in patients' TIL as compared to its expression in normal peripheral blood T cells (Fig. 4). The expression of some V β genes in HCC TIL was as high as 33%. As shown in Figure 5, significant

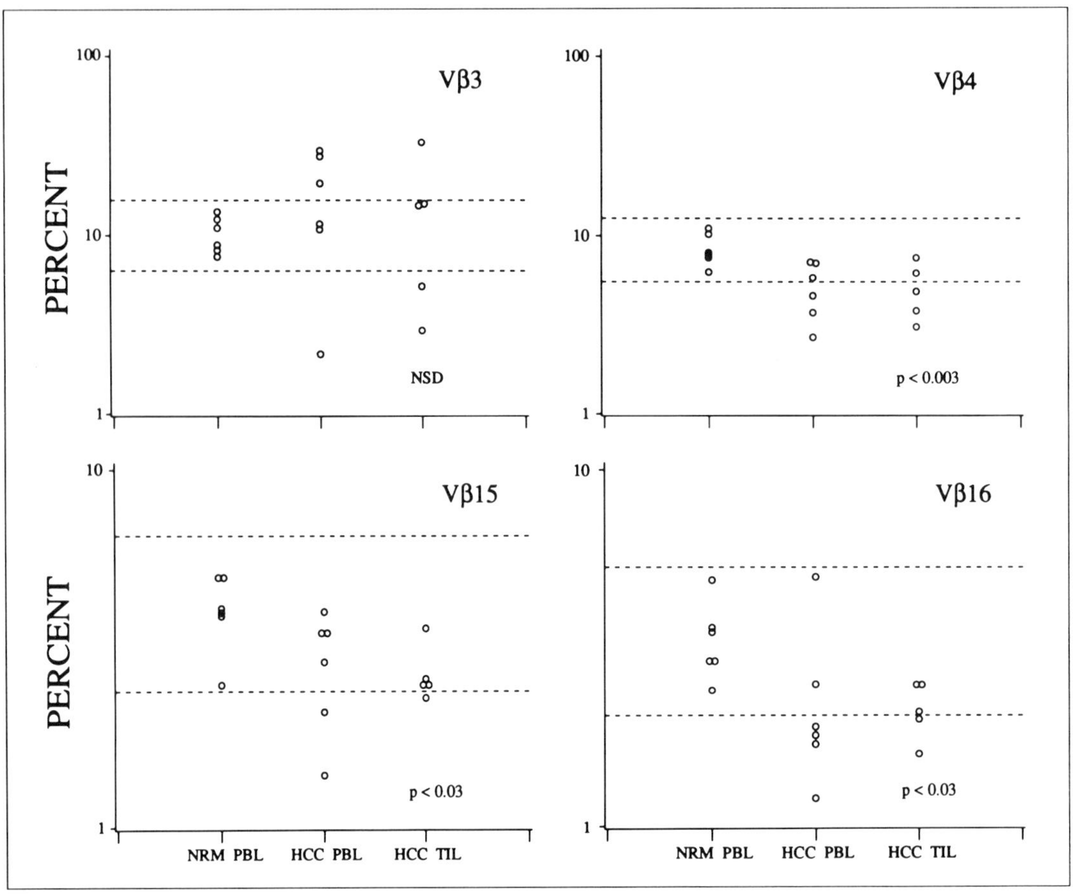

Fig. 5. TcR V β gene expression frequencies were calculated and compared between normal PBL and patients' PBL as well as TIL. Ordinates, percentages of V β gene expression. The frequencies of the TcR V β gene expression for four V β gene families are shown. Note that in some TIL, there was an overexpression and in others, underexpression of the V β genes in comparison to normal (NRM) distribution. Solid vertical lines, normal range; dotted lines, ± 2 SD from the normal mean. Reproduced with permission from Weidmann et al, Cancer Res 1992;52:5913-5920.

differences between control PBL and patients' PBL or TIL were observed for V β-4, V β-15 and V β-16 gene frequencies. Overall, PBL from five out of six cases studied had different V β gene frequencies than those seen in PBL obtained from normal individuals.[59] Thus, not only TIL but also PBL-T in patients with HCC show a restricted usage of certain V β genes, possibly because some of these T cells are involved in immune responses directed at the tumor. Furthermore, when PCR-amplified complementary DNAs of the V β-1 and V β-3 genes obtained from the two TIL preparations were cloned and sequenced by Dr. Weidmann, the same rearrangements were found in the majority of DNA clones.[59] This analysis of TcR V β usage in freshly isolated TIL and in patients' PBL indicated that T lymphocytes in patients with HCC might have restricted immunologic reactivity with respect to AuTu.

More recently, using a quantitative PCR approach we developed earlier, we studied the TcR V β usage of TIL freshly isolated from human metastatic melanomas to test the hypothesis that clones of T cells expressing a particular V β gene may be present among such TIL and might represent AuTu-specific T cells. In addition, expression of the V β genes in T lymphocytes expanded from some of these TIL cultured long-term in the presence of IL-2 and IL-4 was determined. Our results indicated that although fresh TIL obtained from various human melanomas showed oligoclonal expression of certain V β genes (Fig. 6a), the V β repertoire was different in each TIL preparation. Culture of TIL in the presence of IL-2 and IL-4 resulted in in vitro selection and outgrowth of T-cell lines, each expressing the restricted number of TcR V β genes, which were distinct from those preferentially expressed in fresh TIL (Fig. 6b). These selected T-cell lines were $CD3^+CD8^+$ in early TIL cultures, and expression of a restricted number of the V β genes by these lines did not seem to correlate with the presence or level of AuTu cytotoxicity mediated by cultured TIL.[58] These recent data indicate that the V β gene usage is restricted in fresh TIL but that the restrictions

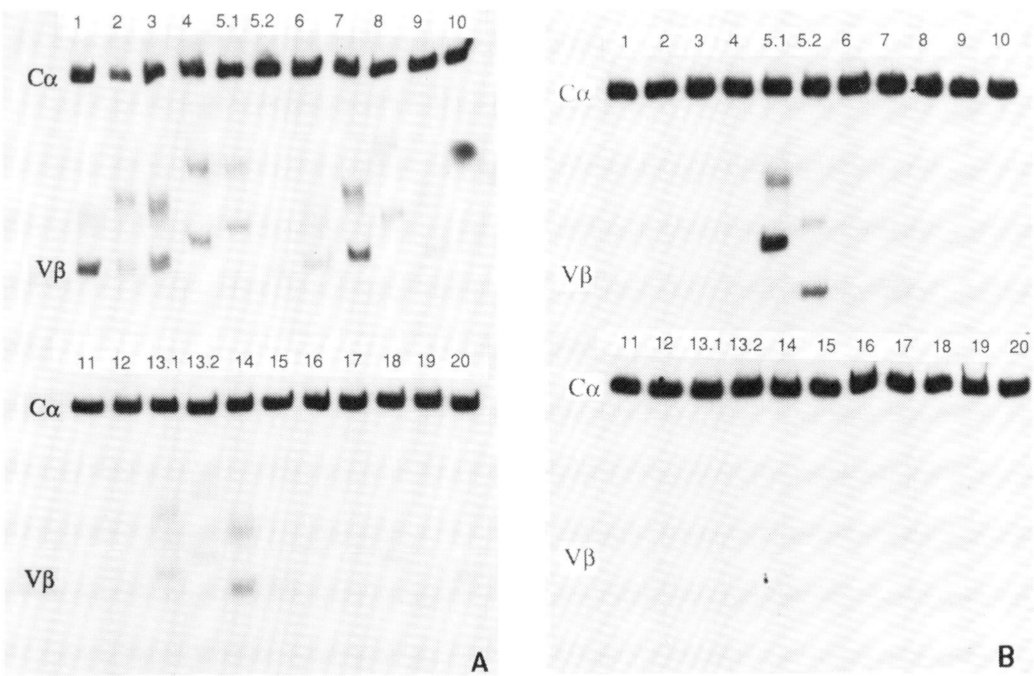

Fig. 6. TcR V β-gene expression in fresh TIL preparation (a). Note expression of V β-1, -2, -3, -5.1 and -7 and absence of V β-10, -11, -15 and -16. The same TIL preparation was cultured in the presence of IL-2 and IL-4. In (b) TcR V β-gene expression on TIL studied on day 60 of growth is shown. Note predominant expression of V β-5.1 and V β-5.2 in cultured TIL. Reproduced with permission from Weidmann et al, Int. J. Cancer 1993; 54:383-390.

are different in every tumor.[59,60] Furthermore, random outgrowth in culture appears to be responsible for selection of T-cell lines expressing the V β genes, which are not prominently expressed by fresh TIL.[59]

SUMMARY

The phenotypic characterization of fresh TIL in suspensions of different human solid tumors by two-color flow cytometry has allowed for a more precise quantitation of T-cell subsets than earlier immunohistologic studies. Also, it has been possible to identify differences between TIL, tumor-involved or -uninvolved lymph nodes and A-PBL by flow cytometry.[4,19,61] On the whole, newer phenotypic data have emphasized the presence of activated or committed T lymphocytes among TIL. The more recent application of three-color or multiparameter flow cytometry to phenotypic analysis of TIL promises to provide more insights into expression of activation markers and adhesion molecules on these cells. Molecular analysis of the TcR V region genes in TIL isolated from several types of tumors indicated that V β gene expression was oligoclonal among TIL and that restrictions in V β gene expression differed among tumors with the same histology.

Improved understanding of the role T cells expressing permanent activation markers in situ play in human solid tumors leads to a consideration that adoptive transfer of tumor-reactive $CD4^+CD29^+CD45RO^+$ lymphocytes may be as beneficial in patients with cancer as that with $CD8^+$ cytotoxic cells. Indeed, Dillman et al[62] reported a favorable clinical response in a patient who was treated with in vitro activated TIL with $CD4^+$ phenotype, and 8 of 11 patients treated with TIL at the Surgery Branch, NCI, who showed a partial or mixed response received cells containing >80% $CD4^+$ cells.[63] Such in vitro Ag-activated $CD4^+$ populations might be able to reach tumor deposits, recruit other immune cells to the site and provide helper function locally. It is also possible that RANTES or other cytokines perhaps of the sis-protein superfamily could be valuable components of such transfer, facilitating a selective influx of $CD4^+CD29^+CD45RO^+$ or even $CD8^+CD29^+CD45RO^+$ cells into the tumor.[64,65] Therapeutic effectiveness of IVS LNL in ongoing IVS protocols[66,67] may be perhaps explained in terms of beneficial local contributions of tumor Ag-primed $CD4^+$ lymphocytes.

REFERENCES

1. Pretlow TP, Pretlow TG. Cell Separation: Methods and Selected Applications. New York:Academic Press, 1986.
2. Whiteside TL, Miescher S, MacDonald RH, Von Fliedner V. Separation of tumor-infiltrating lymphocytes from tumor cells in human solid tumors. A comparison between velocity sedimentation and discontinuous density gradients. J Immunol Methods 1986; 90:221-233.
3. Vanky F, Klein E. Autotumor lytic potential of lymphocytes separated from human solid tumors. In: Herberman RB., ed.NK Cells and Other Natural Effector Cells. New York: Academic Press, 1991: 1061-1068.
4. Cardi G, Mastrangelo MJ, Berd D. Depletion of T-cells with the CD4+CD45R+ phenotype in lymphocytes that infiltrate subcutaneous metastases of human melanoma. Cancer Res 1989; 49:6562-6565.
5. Finke JH, Rayman P, Alexander J, Edinger M, Tubbs RR, Connelly R, Pontes E, Bukowski R. Characterization of the cytolytic activity of CD4+ and CD8+ tumor-infiltrating lymphocytes in human renal cell carcinoma. Cancer Res 1990; 50:2363-2370.
6. Bilik R, Mor C, Hazaz B, Moroz C. Characterization of T-lymphocyte subpopulations infiltrating primary breast cancer. Cancer Immunol Immunother 1989; 28:143-147.
7. Rabinowich H, Cohen R, Bruderman I, Steiner Z, Klajman A. Functional analysis of mononuclear cells infiltrating into tumors: lysis of autologous human tumor cells by cultured infiltrating lymphocytes. Cancer Res 1987; 47:173-177.
8. Moore K, Walters MT, Jones DB, Garvey E, Harvey J, Cawley MI, Smith JL. An immunohistological study of CD4+ lymphocyte subsets within inflammatory lesions with special reference to rheumatoid arthritis and inflammatory bowel disease. Immunol 1988; 65:457-463.

9. Pitzalis C, Kingsley G, Haskard D, Panayi G. The preferential accumulation of helper-inducer T lymphocytes in inflammatory lesions: evidence for regulation by selective endothelial and homotypic adhesion. Eur J Immunol 1988; 18:1397-1404.
10. Vose BM, Moore M. Human tumor-infiltrating lymphocytes: A marker of host response. Semin Hematol 1985; 22:27-40.
11. Kornstein MJ, Brooks JS, Elder DE. Immunoperoxidase localization of lymphocyte subsets in the host response to melanoma and nevi. Cancer Res 1983; 43:2749-2753.
12. Snyderman CH, Heo DS, Chen K, Whiteside TL, Johnson JT. T-cell markers in tumor-infiltrating lymphocytes of head and neck cancer. Head & Neck 1989; 11:331-336.
13. Wolf G, Hudson J, Peterson K, Miller H, McClatchey KD. Lymphocyte subpopulations infiltrating squamous carcinomas of the head and neck: Correlations with extent of tumor and prognosis. Otolaryngol Head Neck Surg 1986; 95:142-152.
14. Heo DS, Whiteside TL, Johnson JT, Chen K, Barnes EL, Herberman RB. Long-term interleukin 2-dependent growth and cytotoxic activity of tumor-infiltrating lymphocytes (TIL) from human squamous cell carcinomas of the head and neck. Cancer Res 1987; 47:6353-6362.
15. Whiteside TL. Human tumor-infiltrating lymphocytes and their characterization. In: Lotzova E, Herberman RB., eds.Role of Interleukin 2 Activated Killer Cells in Cancer. Boca Raton: CRC Press, Inc., 1990: 133-151.
16. Shimizu Y, Iwatsuki S, Herberman RB, Whiteside TL. Clonal analysis of tumor-infiltrating lymphocytes from human primary and metastatic liver tumors. Int J Cancer 1990; 46:878-883.
17. Whitford P, Mallon EA, George WD, Campbell AM. Flow cytometric analysis of tumor-infiltrating lymphocytes in breast cancer. Br J Cancer 1990; 62:971-975.
18. Alexander JP, Kudoh S, Melsop KA, Hamilton TA, Edinger MG, Tubbs RR, Sica D, Tuason L, Klein E, Bukowski RM, Finke JH. T-cells infiltrating renal cell carcinoma display a poor proliferative response even though they can produce interleukin 2 and express interleukin 2 receptors. Cancer Res 1993; 53:1380-1387.
19. Snyderman CH, Heo DS, Johnson JT, d'Amico F, Barnes L, Whiteside TL. Functional and phenotypic analysis of lymphocytes isolated from tumors and lymph nodes of patients with head and neck cancer. Arch Otolaryngol Head Neck Surg 1991; 117:899-905.
20. Sanders ME, Makgoba MW, Shaw S. Human naive and memory T cells: Reinterpretation of helper-inducer and suppressor-inducer subsets. Immunol Today 1988; 9:195-199.
21. Tonks NK, Charbonneau H, Diltz CD, Fischer EH, Walsh KA. Demonstration that the leukocyte common antigen CD45 is a protein tyrosine phosphatase. Biochemistry 1988; 27:8695-8701.
22. Streuli M, Hall LR, Saga Y, Schlossman SF, Saito H. Differential usage of three exons generates at least five different mRNAs encoding human leukocyte common antigens. J Exp Med 1987; 166:1548-1566.
23. Thomas ML, Lefrancois L. Differential expression of the leucocyte-common antigen family. Immunol Today 1988; 9:320-326.
24. Morimoto C, Letvin NL, Distaso JA, Aldrich WR, Schlossman SF. The isolation and characterization of the human suppressor inducer T-cell subset. J Immunol 1985; 134:1508-1515.
25. Smith SH, Brown MH, Rowe D, Callard RE, Beverley PC. Functional subsets of human helper-inducer cells defined by a new monoclonal antibody, UCHL1. Immunol 1986; 58:63-70.
26. Morimoto C, Letvin NL, Boyd AW, Hagan M, Brown HM, Kornacki MM, Schlossman SF. The isolation and characterization of the human helper inducer T-cell subset. J Immunol 1985; 134:3762-3769.
27. Serra HM, Krowka JF, Ledbetter JA, Pilarski LM. Loss of CD45R (Lp220) represents a post-thymic T-cell differentiation event. J Immunol 1988; 140:1435-1441.
28. Akbar AN, Terry L, Timms A, Beverley PC, Janossy G. Loss of CD45R and gain of UCHL1 reactivity is a feature of primed T cells. J Immunol 1988; 140:2171-2178.
29. Clement LT, Yamashita N, Martin AM. The functionally distinct subpopulations of human CD4+ helper/inducer T lymphocytes

defined by anti-CD45R antibodies derive sequentially from a differentiation pathway that is regulated by activation-dependent-post-thymic differentiation. J Immunol 1988; 141:1464-1470.
30. Whiteside TL, Jost LM, Herberman RB. Tumor-infiltrating lymphocytes: Potential and limitations to their use for cancer therapy. Crit Rev Oncol /Hematol 1992; 25-47.
31. Alexander J, Connelly R, Edinger M, Tubbs R, Boyett J, Pontes E, Murthy S, Bukowski R, Finke J. Tumor-infiltrating lymphocytes from renal cell carcinoma: State of activation, phenotypes and functional analysis. Proc AACR 1990; 31:254-A1505.
32. Alexander J, Rayman P, Edinger M, Connelly R, Tubbs R, Bukowski R, Pontes E, Finke J. TIL from renal-cell carcinoma: Restimulation with tumor influences proliferation and cytolytic activity. Int J Cancer 1990; 45:119-124.
33. Modlin RL, Melancon-Kaplan J, Young SM, Pirmez C, Kino H, Convit J, Rea TH, Bloom BR. Learning from lesions: patterns of tissue inflammation in leprosy. PNAS USA 1988; 85:1213-1217.
34. Pirmez C, Cooper C, Paes-Oliveira M, Schubach A, Torigian VK, Modlin RL. Immunologic responsiveness in American cutaneous leishmaniasis lesions. J Immunol 1990; 145:3100-3104.
35. Poulter LW, Duke O, Panayi GS, Hobbs S, Raftery MJ, Janossy G. Activated T lymphocytes of the synovial membrane in rheumatoid arthritis and other arthropathies. Scand J Immunol 1985; 22:683-690.
36. Hemler ME, Glass D, Coblyn JS, Jacobson JG. Very late activation antigens on rheumatoid synovial fluid T lymphocytes. Association with stages of T-cell activation. J Clin Invest 1986; 78:696-702.
37. Kingsley G, Pitzalis C, Kyriazis N, Panayi GS. Abnormal helper-inducer/suppressor-inducer T-cell subset distribution and T-cell activation status are common to all types of chronic synovitis. Scand J Immunol 1988; 28:225-232.
38. Saltini C, Kirby M, Trapnell BC, Tamura N, Crystal RG. Biased accumulation of T lymphocytes with "memory"-type CD45 leukocyte common antigen gene expression on the epithelial surface of the human lung. J Exp Med 1990; 171:1123-1140.
39. Barnes PF, Mistry SD, Cooper CL, Pirmez C, Rea TH, Modlin RL. Compartmentalization of a CD4+ T lymphocyte subpopulation in tuberculous pleuritis. J Immunol 1989; 142:1114-1119.
40. Dvorak HF, Galli SJ, Dvorak AM. Expression of cell-mediated hypersensitivity in vivo: Recent advances. Int Rev Exp Pathol 1980; 21:119-194.
41. Wedmore CV, Williams TJ. Control of vascular permeability by polymorphonuclear leukocytes in inflammation. Nature 1981; 289:646-650.
42. Hanto DW, Hopt UT, Hoffman R, Simmons RL. Lymphocyte recruitment, regional blood flow, and vascular permeability at sites of allogeneic cellular interactions. J Immunol 1982; 129:2437-2443.
43. Stoolman LM. Adhesion molecules controlling lymphocyte migration. Cell 1989; 56:907-910.
44. Damle NK, Doyle LV. Stimulation of cloned human T lymphocytes via the CD3 or CD28 molecules induces enhancement in vascular endothelial permeability to macromolecules with participation of type-1 and type-2 intercellular adhesion pathways. Eur J Immunol 1990; 20:1995-2003.
45. Vujanovic NL, Herberman RB, Olszowy MW, Cramer DV, Salup RR, Reynolds CW, Hiserodt JC. Lymphokine-activated killer cells in rats: Analysis of progenitor and effector cell phenotype and relationship to natural killer cells. Cancer Res 1988; 48:884-890.
46. Vaccarello L, Kanbour A, Kanbour-Shakir A, Whiteside TL. Tumor-infiltrating lymphocytes from ovarian tumors of low malignant potential. Int J Gynecol Pathol 1993; 12:41-50.
47. Moy PM, Holmes EC, Golub SH. Depression of natural killer cytotoxic activity in lymphocytes infiltrating human pulmonary tumors. Cancer Res 1985; 45:57-60.
48. Zocchi MR, Ferrarini M, Rugarli C. Selective lysis of the autologous tumor by δ TCS1+ γ/δ+ tumor-infiltrating lymphocytes from human lung carcinomas. Eur J Immunol 1990; 20:2685-2689.

49. Nanno M, Seki H, Mathioudakis G, Suzuki R, Itoh K, Ioannides CG, Suzuki S, Chen PF, Platsoucas CD. γ/δ T-cell antigen receptors expressed on tumor-infiltrating lymphocytes from patients with solid tumors. Eur J Immunol 1992; 22:679-687.
50. Ferrarini M, Heltai S, Zocchi R, Rugarli C. Unusual expression and localization of heat-shock proteins in human tumor cells. Int J Cancer 1992; 51:613-619.
51. Oksenberg JR, Stuart S, Begovich AB, Bell RB, Ehrlich HA, Steinman L, Bernard CCA. Limited heterogeneity of rearranged T-cell-receptor V α transcripts in brains of multiple sclerosis patients. Nature (London) 1990; 345:344-348.
52. Paliard X, West SG, Lafferty JA, Clements JR, Kappler J, Marrack P, Kotzin BL. Evidence for the effects of a superantigen in rheumatoid arthritis. Science 1991; 253:325-329.
53. Hafler DA, Duby AD, Lee SJ, Benjamin D, Sideman JG, Weiner HL. Oligoclonal T lymphocytes in the cerebrospinal fluid of patients with multiple sclerosis. J Exp Med 1988; 167:1313-1322.
54. Posnett DN, Schmelkin L, Bruton DA, August A, McGrath H, Mayer LF. T-cell antigen receptor V gene usage increases in V β+ T cells in Crohn's disease. J Clin Invest 1990; 85:1770-1776.
55. Nitta T, Oksenberg JR, Rao NA, Steinman L. Predominant expression of T-cell receptor V α 7 in tumor-infiltrating lymphocytes of uveal melanoma. Science 1990; 249:672-674.
56. Karpati RM, Banks SM, Malissen B, Rosenberg SA, Sheard MA, Weber JS, Hodes RJ. Phenotypic characterization of murine tumor-infiltrating T lymphocytes. J Immunol 1991; 146:2043-2051.
57. Ioannides CG, Freedman RS. Selective usage of TcR V β in tumor-specific CTL lines isolated from ovarian tumor-associated lymphocytes. AntiCancer Res 1991; 11:1919-1925.
58. Weidmann E, Elder EM, Trucco M, Lotze MT, Whiteside TL. Usage of T-cell receptor V β chain genes in fresh and cultured tumor-infiltrating lymphocytes from human melanoma. Int J Cancer 1993; 54:383-390.
59. Weidmann E, Whiteside TL, Giorda R, Herberman RB, Trucco M. The T-cell receptor V β gene usage in tumor-infiltrating lymphocytes and blood of patients with hepatocellular carcinoma. Cancer Res 1992; 52:5913-5920.
60. Nitta T, Sato K, Okumura K, Steinman L. An analysis of T-cell-receptor variable-region genes in tumor-infiltrating lymphocytes within malignant tumors. Int J Cancer 1991; 49:545-550.
61. Shimizu Y, Iwatsuki S, Herberman RB, Whiteside TL. Effects of cytokines on in vitro growth of tumor-infiltrating lymphocytes obtained from human primary and metastatic liver tumors. Cancer Immunol Immunother 1991; 32:280-288.
62. Dillman RO, Oldham RK, Birch R, Barth NM, Cohen RJ, Minor DR, Maleckar J, Yannelli J, West WW. Treatment of melanoma with interleukin-2 (IL-2) and tumor-derived activated cells (TDAC). Proc Am Soc Clin Oncol 1990; 9:276-A1069.
63. Rosenberg SA, Packard BS, Aebersold PM, Solomon D, Topalian SL, Toy ST, Simon P, Lotze MT, Yang JC, Seipp CA, Simpson C, Carter C, Bock S, Schwartzentruber D, Wei JP, White DE. Use of tumor-infiltrating lymphocytes and interleukin-2 in the immunotherapy of patients with metastatic melanoma. A preliminary report. N Engl J Med 1988; 319:1676-1680.
64. Schall TJ, Jongstra J, Dyer BJ, Jorgensen J, Clayberger C, Davis MM, Krensky AM. A human T-cell-specific molecule is a member of a new gene family. J Immunol 1988; 141:1018-1025.
65. Schall TJ, Bacon K, Toy KJ, Goeddel DV. Selective attraction of monocytes and T lymphocytes of the memory phenotype by cytokine RANTES. Nature 1990; 347:669-671.
66. Logan T, Kirkwood J, Wolmark N, Whiteside T, Elder E, Vlock D, Ernstoff M, Dexter L, Posner M, Herberman R. Pilot study of in vitro sensitized T cells in adoptive transfer therapy of cancer. Proc Am Soc Clin Oncol 1990; 9:188-A726.
67. Chang AE, Yoshizawa H, Sakai K, Cameron MJ, Sondak VK, Shu S. Clinical observations on adoptive immunotherapy with vaccine-primed T lymphocytes secondarily sensitized to tumor in vitro. Cancer Res 1993; 53:1043-1050.

CHAPTER 5

Functional Characteristics of Fresh TIL

Functional studies of TIL freshly obtained from human tumors have been difficult to perform due mainly to a limited number of cells and the presence of tumor cells in the final TIL preparations. It has been suggested in the past that the possibility of selective losses, which might occur during TIL separation from tissue, precludes adequate functional assessment of fresh TIL. Similarly, enzymatic treatments were thought to have a negative effect on functions of fresh TIL, until responses of TIL processed with and without enzymatic digestion were compared and found to be identical.[1-3] In general, functional assessments of human TIL have been performed following activation and expansion of TIL in culture, and few studies of fresh TIL performed immediately after their isolation from tumor are available.[4,5] Yet, it has been largely due to these few studies that a functional deficit of TIL in situ has been identified[6] and confirmed in more recent experiments.[7] It is obvious that TIL present in the tumor are not effective in controlling disease in vivo. As discussed earlier, tumors progress even though they contain considerable infiltrates of T lymphocytes. In this chapter, evidence for impaired functional responses of TIL will be reviewed, and an attempt will be made to explain the possible reasons for this deficiency.

LIMITATIONS OF FUNCTIONAL STUDIES WITH TIL

The small number of TIL available after their isolation from tumor and purification has restricted the use of standard immunologic assays for assessment of TIL. Only more recently, with the introduction of micromethods, simultaneous assessment of several functional parameters has become possible with fresh TIL. The main remaining obstacle has been the presence of tumor cells in many TIL preparations following enrichment. The presence of nonlymphoid cells among TIL is undesirable because of the possibility that these cells may interfere with the interpretation of results or may contribute to the frequently observed deficiency in functional responses of TIL. In vitro assays of TIL functions generally require AuTu cells as a source of stimulatory Ags, as targets for cytotoxicity assays or for monitoring of cytokine production in response to AuTu. Fresh tumor cells with good viability and purity satisfactory for these assays are often not available or not recovered in the adequate number. An alternative approach is to establish tumor cell lines, but tissue culture of tumor cells is both time-consuming and often unsuccessful. Another limitation, which has tended to bias the interpretation of TIL function, is the fact that human TIL are almost invariably recovered from advanced tumors. In very few instances were fresh TIL recovered from premalignant, early malignant or adjacent noninvolved tissues and characterized functionally. Frequent functional comparisons have been made between TIL and A-PBL or normal PBL, although clearly, it would be more informative to compare TIL and tissue lymphocytes from benign lesions or chronic inflammatory infiltrates in the same anatomic location as that of the tumor which is the source of TIL. Although TIL obtained from primary tumors vs. tumor metastases have been functionally assessed, longitudinal studies of human TIL comparable to those of murine TIL are not possible, unless immunotherapy is instituted and serial biopsies are available to evaluate response. Despite the limitations listed above, freshly isolated TIL from a variety of human tumors have been functionally evaluated and found to have impaired proliferative and cytotoxic responses.

PROLIFERATION AND CYTOTOXICITY OF FRESHLY ISOLATED TIL

Functional unresponsiveness of some human TIL was first observed in the early 1980s, when freshly isolated TIL preparations were examined for proliferation and antitumor cytotoxicity in vitro.[5] These early studies indicated that freshly isolated TIL exhibit the following characteristics: (a) poor cytotoxic activity against AuTu or allogeneic NK-sensitive or NK-resistant tumor cell targets;[8-12] (b) decreased ability to proliferate in response to mitogens or allogeneic stimulators in mixed lymphocyte culture;[1,2,6,13,14] and (c) capability to suppress the mitogen and tumor-induced proliferation as well as LAK activity of autologous blood lymphocytes.[15,16] In contrast to TIL, PBL of patients with cancer often show normal responsiveness in assays of cytotoxicity, natural killing, and proliferation.[11,17] In fact, it has been shown that PBL may be a better source of antitumor effector cells than TIL in mixed lymphocyte tumor cultures (MLTC).[18-23]

Several years ago, we compared in vitro responses to IL-2 and allogeneic lymphocytes of TIL and A-PBL in patients with various tumors.[6] Our results indicated that TIL were uniformly unresponsive to mitogens and phorbol ester and often unable to proliferate in response to IL-2. Furthermore, responses of TIL in MLC were often depressed as compared with A-PBL.[6] Alexander and colleagues have also examined responses of TIL obtained from human RCC to anti-CD3 mAb and IL-2 or IL-2 alone and compared them to those of A-PBL.[7] Their results confirmed proliferative unresponsiveness of fresh TIL, as compared with A-PBL. That TIL-T are intrinsically unable to respond to exogenous activation stimuli, has been convincingly demonstrated by Miescher and collaborators.[13,14] Sorted $CD2^+$ TIL from a variety of solid tumors stimulated by either phytohemagglutinin (PHA)-P or anti-CD3 mAb in low-density cultures were unable to proliferate even though the structurally intact CD3-TcR α/β complex was present on these cells as confirmed by flow cytometry.[14] The depressed proliferative response of these TIL could not be reversed by phorbol esters alone or in combination with ionomycin, which bypass the TcR.[13,14] These experiments showed that the Ag-dependent proliferation pathway was impaired in TIL, and that this impairment was greater among $CD8^+$ than $CD4^+$ TIL subpopulations.[24] It is important to add that in all the above described experiments, Ag-presenting cells (APC) were added to the microcultures of TIL in the form of irradiated A-PBL or autologous adherent monocytes to assure that adequate APC were available. Thus, the observed TIL unresponsiveness appeared to be their intrinsic property and was not due to the absence or functional incompetence of APC.

The additional confirmation of a functional defect in freshly isolated TIL came from studies that compared the clonogenic potential of TIL to that of A-PBL using limiting dilution analysis (LDA) in several types of human solid tumors.[1,2,6,25,26] This type of analysis showed that the clonogenic potential of TIL-T was significantly reduced in comparison to T cells obtained from A-PBL or normal PBL (see Fig. 1).[1,6] The LDA permitted calculations of the frequency of proliferating T lymphocyte precursors (PTL-p) among TIL. In LDA performed with TIL obtained from different types of solid tumors, only about 1 in 20 T cells was able to proliferate under culture conditions allowing every normal PBL-T to grow.[13,14] Further, this low PTL-p frequency was not due to enzymatic digestion of tumor tissue, as demonstrated repeatedly in experiments performed in our laboratory.[1,6] In both LDA and low-density cultures, $CD8^+$ TIL, separated by sorting from $CD4^+$ TIL were preferentially unresponsive to proliferative stimuli.[24]

Freshly isolated TIL have also been reported to lack or express reduced levels of antitumor cytotoxicity.[9-11,27] This deficiency of TIL has been first demonstrated with bulk TIL[6] and further examined at a clonal level.[2] Clonal analysis of TIL is thought to be important for the demonstration of AuTu-specific CTL, as tumor specific responses mediated by CTL may be difficult to distinguish from LAK activity in IL-2-dependent bulk cultures of TIL. Using LDA followed by cytotoxicity assays of proliferating TIL clones, it was possible to determine frequencies of cytolytic T-cell precursors (CTL-p) in TIL obtained from various tumors.[2] This frequency was highly variable in TIL obtained from different types of tumors, e.g., ranging from <1% to 21% against K562 targets; from <1% to 12% against allogeneic tumor targets, and from <1% to 18% against AuTu in a study of TIL from liver tumors (hepatocellular and cholangiocarcinomas as well as gastric and colon carcinomas metastatic to

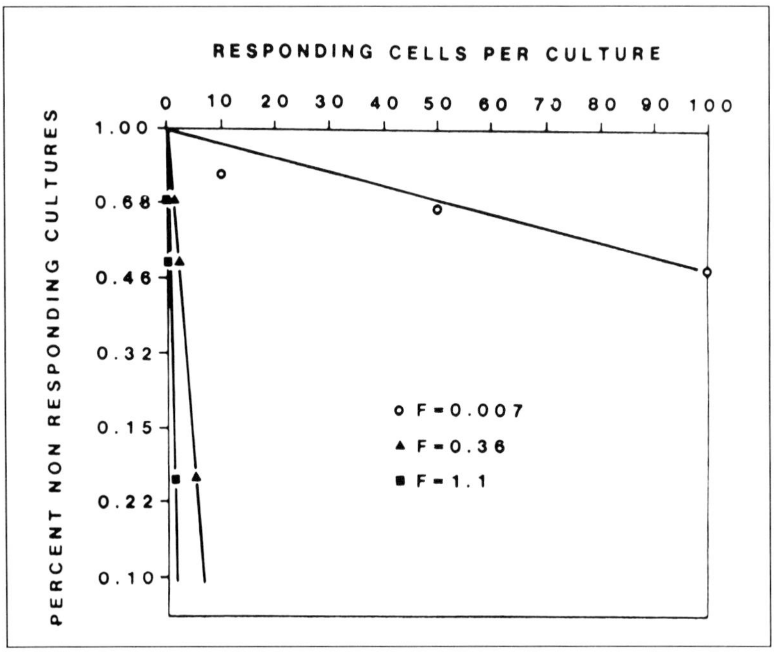

Fig. 1. Limiting dilution analysis of the frequency (F) of proliferating cells obtained from a patient with breast carcinoma: TIL-T o—o, autologous PBL-T ▲—▲ and normal PBL-T ■—■ Cells were plated according to the number of $CD2^+$ T lymphocytes at varying cell doses per well in the presence of irradiated feeder cells. 1% PHA (v/v), and an exogenous source of IL-2. After 14-25 days of culture, each well was scored microscopically for proliferation. Each point is based on a minimum of 42 microcultures. The regression line was fitted to the data by the minimum χ^2 method. Reproduced with permission from Whiteside et al, Cancer Immunol Immunother 1986; 23:163-178.

liver) performed in our laboratory.[26] Of course, these clones of TIL were cultured in the presence of IL-2 and irradiated feeder cells prior to cytotoxicity assays.[2,26] At the same time, CTL-p against AuTu were identified only in TIL and were not found among cells from A-PBL in our study, indicating that TIL contain CTL-p against AuTu.[26] When clones of TIL were tested in lectin-dependent cellular cytotoxicity (LDCC) assays, which allow detection of a cytolytic potential irrespective of antigenic specificity of effector cells, as the lectin acts by triggering the cytotoxic machinery via the TcR, it was possible to conclude that TIL possess a significant cytotoxic potential.[25] A majority of the growing microcultures (up to 67%) from TIL preparations had a cytolytic potential, as based on results of LDCC, while LAK activity was only infrequently observed.[25] The most interesting finding was that many CD4$^+$/CD8$^-$ clones (which, in most cases, represented a majority of proliferating TIL) generated from TIL were capable of mediating LDCC.[25] Only a small proportion (<5%) of CD4$^+$ clones from normal PBL or PBL of cancer patients mediate LDCC (see Fig. 2). It can be concluded from this observation that at least some human tumors contain CD4$^+$ T lymphocyte precursors with the cytolytic potential. Equally interesting is the relative paucity of CD8$^+$ T-cell clones outgrowing from TIL preparations as compared to T cells obtained from normal or A-PBL and cultured under the same experimental conditions.[25] It is reasonable to conclude that fresh TIL, which contain mixtures of CD8$^+$ and CD4$^+$ T cells, have depressed proliferative responses to a variety of stimuli, and that CD4$^+$ TIL proliferate preferentially. Those TIL that do proliferate in vitro have a cytolytic potential which is not restricted to CD8$^+$ T cells and encompasses CD4$^+$ T cells as well.

One of the most important observations which has emerged from functional studies of TIL relates to differences observed between TIL obtained from primary tumors as compared to those obtained from tumor metastases. Our recent results have shown that fresh TIL from primary liver tumors, especially hepatocellular carcinoma, were a significantly better source of antitumor effector cells than those obtained from hepatic metastases of colon tumors, with the latter showing cytotoxicity against AuTu in only 1/66 clones established from fresh TIL.[26] In spite of this low frequency of AuTu-reactive CTL-p in colon tumors metastatic to liver, we were successful in obtaining several AuTu-specific, cytolytic T-cell clones (CD3$^+$CD8$^+$) from TIL of gastric carcinoma metastasized into liver.[26,28]

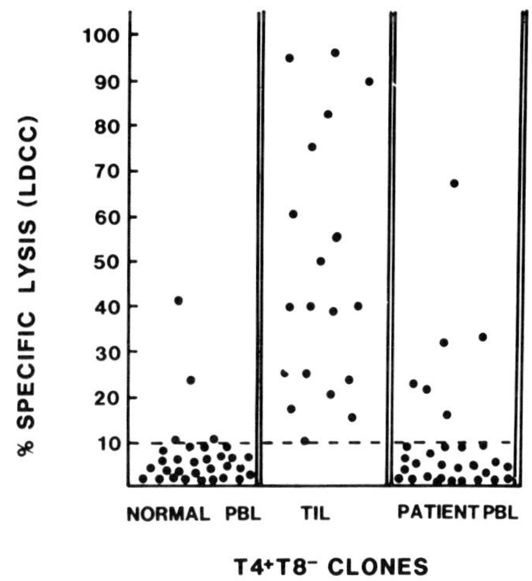

Fig. 2. Comparison of cytolytic activities in lectin-dependent cellular cytotoxicity assays of randomly selected T4$^+$/T8$^-$ clones derived from normal PBL, TIL from breast carcinomas and PBL from patients with breast tumors. The dotted line represents 3 SD over background values given by the spontaneous release of ^{51}Cr-labeled P815 targets. Reproduced with permission from Whiteside et al, Cancer Immunol Immunother 1986; 23:163-178.

OTHER FUNCTIONS OF FRESHLY ISOLATED TIL

In addition to proliferation and cytotoxicity, another function of lymphocytes, that of locomotion, has been recently described to be deficient in TIL obtained from human melanoma and RCC.[29] Locomotion of fresh TIL was investigated in vitro using a three-dimensional collagen gel model. TIL migration was found to be completely inhibited compared with migration of normal and cancer patient peripheral blood leukocytes and lymphocytes from lymph nodes. Long-term culture of TIL in 200 U/ml of IL-2 reinstated locomotor ability, but short-term exposure of TIL to a variety of cytokines had no effect on migration.[29]

The ability of freshly isolated TIL to produce cytokines or to express message for cytokines has been tested recently in a limited number of studies.[7,30] Spontaneous or in vitro-induced production of IL-2 by TIL freshly isolated from patients with HNC were found to be comparable to those of PBL (Table 1) in a recent study performed in our laboratory.[30] In contrast, in vitro-induced production of IFN-γ, TNF-α or IL-1-β was lower in TIL than in PBL (Table 1). Interestingly, spontaneous production of TNF-α or IL-1-β was significantly elevated in PBL of patients with HNC as compared to normal controls. TIL did not show this increase, and their spontaneous cytokine production was similar to that of normal PBL.[30] Our ISH studies for expression of cytokine genes in TIL described in Chapter 2 also suggest that the cytokine induction pathway is intact, at least in TIL from certain breast and SCCHN tumors.[30] A recent analysis performed by Alexander and colleagues of cytokine and cytokine receptor (IL-2R) gene expression linked to the TcR/CD3 or IL-2 stimulation in TIL obtained from RCC has shown that certain signaling pathways associated with these receptors are intact in TIL-T, even in the absence of TIL proliferation in response to PHA or anti-CD3 mAb + IL-2.[7] TIL-T that did not proliferate produced IL-2 and IFN-γ, expressed IL-2R on the cell surface and at the message level, expressed mRNA for these cytokines comparably to PBL.[7] Thus, it seems that if, intrinsic functional deficit exists in TIL, it is selective, being limited to proliferative, and in part, cytolytic responses, but it does not appear to involve signaling pathways associated with the TcR or IL-2R.[7]

Table 1. Spontaneous and induced in vitro production of cytokines by freshly isolated TIL or PBL in patients with head and neck cancer[a]

Cytokine	TIL n = 7		Patient PBL n = 10		Normal PBL n = 30	
	Spont.	Induced	Spont.	Induced	Spont.	Induced
IL-2 (U/ml)	2.3±1.6	43±18	2.5±1.8	20±6.8	0.6±0.2	17±2.3
IFN-γ (U/ml)	0	46±23*	2.1±2.3	76±40*	4.6±1.2	267±31
IL-1-β (pg/ml)	47±26	39±17*	1036±525*	1472±824	32±7	4600±473
TNF-α (pg/ml)	36±19	70±35*	370±173*	610±212	12±3.5	1550±128

[a] TIL or PBL (1 x 10^5/well) were separated from tumor tissue and incubated in tissue culture medium (spontaneous) or medium plus 2 mg PHA or 1 mg LPS (induced) for 24h. Culture supernatants were harvested and assayed for cytokines. Normal PBL were obtained from volunteers. The data are means ± SEM.

* $p<0.01$ vs normal PBL

(From Vitolo et al, JNCI Monographs 1992; 13:203-208)

ACTIVATION OF TIL BY ANTI-CD3 OR ANTI-CD28 MABS

While human TIL may not proliferate or proliferate poorly in response to mitogens or low concentrations of IL-2, solid-phase anti-CD3 mAb has been successfully used by some investigators to activate and grow TIL in culture.[7,31] For example, Schoof and collaborators have assessed eight consecutive tumor cell suspensions for outgrowth of TIL in the presence of IL-2 alone (1,000 U/ml) or anti-CD3 mAb coated on the surface of culture flasks (1 μg/ml). They found that TIL proliferation was significantly ($p<0.05$) enhanced in six out of eight samples when solid-phase anti-CD3 was used to initiate TIL cultures.[31] In two of eight TIL cultures, which failed to proliferate in response to high-dose IL-2, anti-CD3 mAb was able to induce activation and proliferation. Also, TIL activated with anti-CD3 produced IL-2, which was detectable by a CTLL-based biologic assay.[31] This study indicated that alternative signals in the form of CD3-specific antibodies may render TIL responsive to proliferation in the presence of low concentrations of IL-2. The possibility of using solid-phase anti-CD3 mAb in conjunction with IL-2 as a stimulus for activation of TIL and for generation in vitro of class I MHC restricted CTL has also been explored by Alexander et al, using TIL obtained from patients with RCC.[7] However, in the hands of these investigators, stimulation of TIL-T via the TcR/CD3 complex and IL-2R did not induce significant proliferative response, even though TIL expressed both CD3 and IL-2R-β, as determined by flow cytometry.[7]

The studies described above indicated that human TIL may not be easily activated in vitro via the Ag-dependent TcR/CD3 complex.[7,14] It is possible, however, that the Ag-independent pathways of T-cell activation mediated by CD2 or CD28 molecules could function in TIL unresponsive to CD3-mediated signals. To test this hypothesis, Zocchi and colleagues studied in vitro responses of TIL obtained from six primary lung tumors and six RCC.[32] They showed that the CD28-mediated activation pathway was functional in human TIL and that signaling with anti-CD28 mAb induced proliferation, cytokine release and Ca^{++} mobilization. Conversely, these TIL responded poorly to stimulation via CD2. In contrast to A-PBL, signaling via CD28 did not synergize with CD2 signaling in human TIL.[32] TIL could be triggered by anti-CD28 alone, without the need of either anti-CD3 or IL-2, which indicated that CD28 did not merely deliver a costimulatory signal. The reason for preferential responsiveness of TIL to anti-CD28 mAb is not clear. It may be hypothesized that the ligand of CD28 (B7/BB1) is expressed at the tumor site and may be responsible for activation of TIL in situ.

EVALUATION OF IMMUNOCOMPETENCE OF FRESH TIL

The functional deficiencies of TIL described above were not an "all or none" phenomenon. On the contrary, some preparations of fresh TIL retained considerable functional activities, and especially, TIL isolated from primary tumors were often more active than those obtained from tumor metastases.[5,33] Also, as indicated above, not all functions of TIL are defective, in vitro proliferation in response to mitogens, anti-CD3 mAb or IL-2 being the most consistently depressed. It is unclear presently how generalized tumor-induced T-cell anergy is, and whether it extends to all or only selected TIL-T functions. Few studies assessing functional competence of fresh TIL other than their cytolytic or proliferative functions have been performed. Specifically, in vitro lymphokine secretion by fresh human TIL upon AuTu stimulation has not been studied extensively.[30] The levels of lymphokines secreted by fresh TIL should be quantitatively evaluated for differences between, e.g., IL-2 and TNF-α; IL-2 and IFN-γ; or IL-2 and GM-CSF, because in vitro secretion of many different cytokines, but not of IL-2, may be a function of cells other than T cells that may be present in TIL preparations. It has been reported that anergic T cells maintain a somewhat diminished ability to release TNF-α, GM-CSF and IFN-γ, but release no or very low levels of IL-2 upon restimulation with high concentrations of the relevant

Ag.[34,35] Thus, anergic or tolerized T cells, such as TIL presumably are, may still secrete cytokines. Additional studies are needed to determine the ability of freshly isolated TIL to produce cytokines, particularly in response to stimulation by AuTu cells.

The phenomenon of T cell unresponsiveness in the microenvironment of human solid tumors has not yet been extensively investigated. Nevertheless, it deserves attention, particularly with respect to TIL, which by virtue of their extended proximity to the tumor in vivo, are likely to be influenced by tumor-derived products. Some of these products have known immunosuppressive properties.[36-41] It remains unclear whether TIL recovered from all or only some solid tumors are in an anergic state or whether TIL unresponsiveness is short- or long-lived. Alexander et al observed that sorted T cells derived from TIL of patients with RCC did not expand in vitro in the presence of autologous feeder cells, when cultured with IL-2 for one to three weeks.[7] Similarly, we reported that to activate TIL isolated from metastatic lesions, high concentrations of IL-2 (6,000 IU/ml) are usually necessary, while lower concentrations of IL-2 may be sufficient for activation of TIL obtained from primary tumors.[33,42] These results suggest that TIL may vary in the degree of unresponsiveness to exogenous stimuli or that higher proportions of TIL are unresponsive in certain tumors than in others. Also, TIL proliferation as well as the type of proliferating cell seem to depend on the presence and concentration of exogenous IL-2 and other cytokines. In ovarian carcinoma, culture of TIL in the presence of high concentrations of IL-2 (6,000 IU/ml) leads to expansion of NK/LAK populations,[43] while their culture in IL-2 concentrations of <600 IU/ml may lead to the outgrowth of T-cell lines.[44] TIL obtained from metastatic tumors may not only require high IL-2 concentrations but, in general, proliferate less well in culture than TIL from primary tumors.[33,42] Again, this would tend to suggest that TIL may be more anergic in certain tumors than in others, and that this anergic state is reversible upon isolation of TIL and their incubation in the presence of exogenous IL-2. It has been suggested that tumor-induced suppression, operating perhaps through a down-regulatory network of T cells and cytokines, is responsible for TIL-T unresponsiveness (see below).

Several alternative hypotheses have been advanced to account for the lack of immune competence of freshly isolated TIL. These are as follows: (a) elimination or deletion of tumor Ag-reactive T lymphocytes from the tumor microenvironment; (b) selective inactivation of AuTu-reactive T cells; (c) down-regulation of T-cell functions by the immunoregulatory network; (d) inability of cells in the tumor to make cytokines, which are necessary for expression of T-cell functions; and (e) production and secretion by human tumors of immunosuppressive factors.

In respect to the first possibility, elimination or clonal deletion of tumor Ag-reactive T cells appears unlikely. As discussed above, AuTu-reactive T-cell lines or clones have been isolated from various human solid tumors[28,45] or even peripheral blood of patients with cancer.[18,19,46,47] In our own studies, two-color flow cytometry with an extensive panel of mAbs failed to detect any substantial phenotype changes between PBL and TIL in many solid tumors, except for the presence of higher proportions of activated T cells and a decrease in $CD3^-CD56^+$ NK cells in TIL vs. PBL.[5] Of course, these observations do not exclude the possibility that a small population of Ag-reactive $CD3^+$ T cells or APC is absent from TIL. However, the fact that TIL show generalized unresponsiveness to nonspecific stimuli as well as tumor Ag argues against such a selective subset deletion. On the other hand, the absence or selective inactivation of the precursor population of antitumor effector cells might be consistent with these observations.

Functional studies performed with TIL and described above have suggested that AuTu-specific T cells are not only present but are enriched among TIL. This in turn implies that human tumors express unique molecules (TAA) not present in normal tissues and capable of priming T cells. However, under certain conditions, e.g., when defective or incomplete Ag presentation occurs (see below), a state of unresponsiveness may be induced in specific AuTu-responsive T cells. Thus, tumor Ag-mediated inactivation of specific T cells either by high concentrations of Ag in a tumor-bearing host or due to inappropriate Ag presentation may lead to the T-cell unresponsiveness. It is noteworthy that in some aspects, fresh TIL-T isolated from the tumor behave like T cells inactivated by an inadequate or ineffective pathway of Ag presentation. For example, when Ag, APC, and exogenous IL-2 are provided, unresponsiveness of TIL-T is completely reversed.[48,49] Also, the failure of tumor-infiltrating macrophages to release certain cytokines, e.g., IL-1, or to mediate oxidative burst has been well documented in the literature.[50,51] Thus the possibility exists that a lack of responsiveness of TIL-T to AuTu by activation and proliferation may be mediated, in part, by poor or absent Ag presentation even though this Ag is presumably present in excessive amounts. On the other hand, TIL-T do not behave exactly as the T cells in a classical state of anergy.[33] Anergized T cells do not proliferate or produce IL-2 when stimulated via the TcR, although they remain responsive to IL-2.[35] In contrast, TIL from RCC produced IL-2 when stimulated via the TcR but failed to proliferate in response to IL-2 or other stimuli.[7]

Tumor-related activation of lymphoid suppressor cells has been proposed as a major mechanism responsible for depressed immunocompetence in patients with cancer.[52] Activation of suppressor circuits is likely to occur in the case of immunogenic tumors which, by virtue of being able to induce antitumor responses, may activate down-regulatory (suppressor) cells. Mukherji and collaborators have extensively analyzed the phenomenon of cell-mediated suppression in vitro and its contribution to regulation of T-cell responses to AuTu.[16,47] A comprehensive analysis of suppressor cell function in tumor-bearing hosts can be found elsewhere.[53] However, we have not been able to demonstrate the presence of lymphoid suppressor cells in some human solid tumors.[54] For example, in patients with HNC, we have used phenotypic and functional assays to search for lymphoid suppressor cells in tumor-involved as well as tumor-uninvolved lymph nodes, but have failed to demonstrate their presence, even though lymph node lymphocytes (LNL) were unable to mediate tumor-directed responses in the autologous system.[54] Neither activation with IL-2 or Con A nor separation of LNL into $CD4^+$ and $CD8^+$ subpopulations and their activation in culture for up to three weeks resulted in in vitro generation of functionally-demonstrable suppressor activity from LNL.[54] Thus, the evidence for tumor-induced activation of the immunoregulatory network remains unconfirmed for most human solid tumors with the exception of malignant melanoma.[47]

Cytokines are short-lived mediators and both in vivo and in vitro cytokine consumption may lead to misleading conclusions about the ability of human TIL to secrete lymphokines. It has been suggested that both production and availability of cytokines in the tumor microenvironment may be limited, possibly because of decreased production by immunosuppressed TIL, but also by excessive consumption of IL-2 or other cytokines by activated "suppressor cells" or by tumor cells which, in some cases, have been shown to express IL-2R.[55,56] This hypothesis has not been extensively investigated, but more recent experiments using ISH with radiolabeled cDNA probes for cytokines demonstrated that in some tumors TIL did not express mRNA for various cytokines.[57] Similarly, in vitro cytokine production by tumor-involved or uninvolved lymph node lymphocytes of patients with HNC was shown to be absent.[54] On the other hand, in other human solid tumors, especially in tumors with large MNC infiltrates, numerous cells positive for cytokine mRNA were detected.[57,58] Further, TIL from several tumors were able produce IL-2 and IFN-γ and express mRNA for these cytokines.[7,30] Thus, evidence for the ability of TIL to produce cytokines in the tumor microenvironment is not complete and more work is needed in this area. In this respect, it should be emphasized that in situ technologies are preferable for functional TIL characterization because of the possibility that a selective loss of lymphoid populations may occur during the process of TIL separation from tumor tissues.

There is a general agreement that human solid tumors may secrete immunosuppressive substances. A large body of literature exists on soluble mediators secreted by different tumors,[36-41] of which several are known to cause impaired lymphocyte responses to mitogens and/or Ags.[36,59,60] Exposure of PBL to supernatants (SNs) of certain tumor cells, but not normal tissue cells such as fibroblasts, renders lymphocytes unresponsive to proliferative stimuli.[6,61] In general, secretion of these factors by tumor cells is demonstrated by testing the ability of SNs of cultured tumor cells to inhibit lymphocyte activation in vitro. Neutralization of immunosuppression mediated by tumor cell SNs can be documented with mAbs specific for, e.g., TGF-β or TGF-α.[59] The balance between Ag recognition, proliferation, and cytokine production required for manifestation of antitumor immune responses in vivo is probably disturbed by immunosuppressive factors present in the tumor microenvironment. These factors may be produced not only by the tumors, but also by the host tissues or even by the TIL themselves.[30]

The functional definition of suppression may vary according to conditions of each experimental assay and a particular tumor system. For example, TGF-β is well-known as a potent inhibitor of lymphocyte proliferation and cytotoxicity.[59,60] However, in the presence of immobilized anti-CD3 mAb, TGF-β exerts a costimulatory effect on T-cell proliferation, which is independent of the IL-2 and IL-2R pathways.[62] Another example of the complexity of the suppressor circuits in tumor recognition by T cells is illustrated by the reported effects of TNF-α on TIL obtained from human tumors. For example, addition of TNF-α to TIL cultured in IL-2 leads to preferential outgrowth of $CD8^+$ cells, more restricted target specificity, and up-regulation of IL-2R on TIL.[63-65] These effects may be interpreted as a reversal of TGF-β-induced suppression. However, some ovarian tumors secrete TNF-α,[66] which may function as a paracrine growth factor. Therefore, in certain instances, TNF-α may increase the tumor mass leading eventually to Ag-specific inactivation of immune effector cells, as discussed above. In general, tumor progression and metastasis at distant sites are facilitated by organ-derived growth factors.[67] Such factors may, in fact, control the process of organ repair and may affect the proliferation of tumor cells. For example, TGF-α may function as a physiological regulator of liver regeneration,[68] and TGF-β may control hepatocyte replication.[69] Such factors, and others, released by host organs following injury, are known to inhibit lymphocyte activation and function.

INTERACTIONS BETWEEN TUMOR AND TIL IN TUMOR MICROENVIRONMENT

Current evidence from both animal experiments and clinical studies indicates that various events that take place at the tumor site or sites of tumor metastasis are regulated by soluble products, cytokines, released in part by tumor cells, in part by infiltrating MNC and in part by stromal or other tissue cells present in the tumor microenvironment. It is quite likely that these mutual interactions determine functions of TIL in situ and consequently both prognosis and disease outcome. This hypothesis emphasizes the heterogeneity of the tumor microenvironment, and it implies that modification of this microenvironment by exogenous biologic agents may be crucial for successful therapy of cancer. Further, biologic or any other modification of the tumor in situ has to be chosen and delivered not haphazardly but carefully and purposefully, and it may have to be specifically tailored to each tumor or its metastases.

Understanding of interactions between TIL and tumor is, therefore, essential for devising novel and more effective cancer therapies. As indicated earlier, many human tumors or metastases are surrounded by infiltrates of $CD3^+$ T cells and macrophages, which are functionally defective.[4] This poor functional performance of infiltrating immune cells in the tumor microenvironment has been considered by some to be responsible for tumor progression, while the failure of immune cells to eliminate metastases, for dissemination of disease. Since in situ functions of TIL appear to determine their antitumor effectiveness, there has been a great deal of interest in the mechanisms involved in unresponsiveness of TIL. Attempts have been made to determine the intracellular pathways involved in TIL signaling via the TcR/CD3 complex. Human TIL do not appear to differ from PBL in surface expression of the TcR, CD3 or IL-2R with respect to the proportion of positive cells or intensity of expression or individual cells.[7] It is likely however, that like murine T lymphocytes obtained from animals bearing tumors for longer than 26 days, $CD8^+$ T cells from cancer patients have alterations or defects in signal transduction.[70,71] In mice bearing colon carcinoma MCA-38, $CD8^+$ T cells were found to have impaired cytotoxicity, decreased expression of TNF-α and granzyme B genes, and decreased ability to mediate antitumor response(s) in vivo as compared to T cells obtained from normal mice or mice bearing tumor for <21 days.[70] T lymphocytes from long-term tumor bearing mice expressed TcR that contained low amounts of CD3-γ and completely lacked the CD3 ζ chain, which was replaced by the Fc epsilon γ chain.[71] In addition, expression of the tyrosine kinases $p56^{lck}$ and $p59^{fyn}$ was also reduced.[71] Similar changes have been observed in TIL from human RCC (J.H. Finke, personal communication). It is likely that these or similar alterations in the TcR and signal transduction pathways are the basis of immune defects in tumor-bearing hosts. It remains to be seen to what extent PBL in cancer patients are affected, and the source as well as nature of factors inducing these defects need to be identified. Immunosuppressive activities of tumor cells are likely to affect functions of TIL to a greater extent than those of PBL-T.

While tumor-mediated immunosuppression has been well documented in the literature,[72,73] the ability of tumors to activate immune effector cells has received relatively little attention. In vitro evidence comes largely from early MLTC studies with freshly isolated human effector cells, TIL, LNL, PBL, cocultured in the presence of irradiated AuTu cells without IL-2 or with SNs containing natural IL-2, in order to achieve outgrowth of T cells able to recognize and lyse AuTu cells.[18,19,74] Clearly, in some human MLTCs, notably those set up with cells obtained from patients with melanoma, it was possible to generate such T cells, although their AuTu-specificity has not been rigorously determined in those early days.[19] More recently, we have provided evidence that NK-resistant tumor cells, such as human SCCHN incubated with highly purified human resting NK cells were able to induce message for cytokines, up-regulate expression of activation markers on the surface of NK cells, increase the ability of these cells to proliferate in the absence of IL-2 and to mediate antitumor cytotoxicity.[75] Furthermore, SCCHN cell lines have been recently found to produce soluble factors stimulatory for human T cells, specifically $CD4^+$ T lymphocytes.[76] Incubation of purified $CD4^+$ cells in the presence of these SNs and in the absence of IL-2 has led to activation, proliferation in 9-day cultures, as well as up-regulation of cytotoxicity and cytokine production in human T cells.[76] These and other studies[76-79] show that human tumors are capable of producing immunostimulatory factors which may play an important role in modulating functional responses of MNC present at the tumor site.

SUMMARY

Functional studies with human TIL and interpretation of results are complicated by differences between tumors in histology, local environment at the site of tumor growth, duration of tumor growth, and intrinsic immunogenicity of each tumor. All of these factors might contribute to phenotypic and functional heterogeneity of cellular infiltrate accumulating in or around tumors. Although it is difficult to generalize, sufficient data have accumulated to permit several specific conclusions about functional responses of human TIL, which are listed in Table 2. Currently available evidence supports the hypothesis that human TIL and especially $CD8^+$ TIL have an intrinsic and selective defect in the Ag-dependent activation pathway which leads to proliferation. Other functional activities of TIL, e.g., locomotion and antitumor cytotoxicity may also be impaired, although cytokine production and expression of mRNA for IL-2 or IFN-γ are normal. It appears quite likely that tumor-derived immunoinhibitory factors, which may be distinct in various human tumors, are responsible for this intrinsic defect of TIL. As TIL have normal expression of activation and memory surface markers, it is possible that functional defects in TIL take place after they reach the activated state at the tumor site. Preliminary evidence suggests that like murine T cells from tumor-bearing mice, human TIL have defects in signal transduction mediated via the TcR and tyrosine kinases $p56^{lck}$ and $p59^{fyn}$, and that these abnormalities may be a basis for immune defects in cancer-bearing individuals in general. Interactions between TIL and tumor cells in the tumor microenvironment are complex and may result not only in immunosuppression but also in immunostimulation of TIL. These findings raise the possibility of novel anticancer therapies aimed at the inactivation of suppressor factors in vivo, thus resulting in desirable improvements of the immune-mediated antitumor responses. Some of the tumor-derived immunopotentiating factors may be useful in the future in efforts to up-regulate activities of TIL in situ. At this time, however, approaches that might lead to overcoming or reversing immunosuppressive influences of the tumor microenvironment in vivo have received relatively little attention.

References

1. Whiteside TL, Miescher S, Hurlimann J, Von Fliedner V. Separation, phenotyping and limiting-dilution analysis of T-lymphocytes infiltrating human solid tumors. Int J Cancer 1986; 37:803-811.
2. Miescher S, Whiteside TL, Moretta L, Von Fliedner V. Clonal and frequency analyses of tumor-infiltrating T lymphocytes from human solid tumors. J Immunol 1987; 138:4004-4011.
3. Von Fliedner V, Qiao L, Whiteside TL, Leyvraz S, Barras C, Miescher S. Clonogenic and functional potential of T lymphocytes infiltrating human solid tumors. In: Truitt RL, Gale RP, Bortin MM., eds.Cellular Immunotherapy of Cancer. New York: Alan R. Liss, Inc., 1987: 223-232.
4. Whiteside TL, Jost LM, Herberman RB. Tumor-infiltrating lymphocytes: Potential and limitations to their use for cancer therapy. Crit Rev Oncol /Hematol 1992; 25-47.
5. Whiteside TL. Tumor-infiltrating lymphocytes as antitumor effector cells. Biotherapy 1992; 5:47-61.
6. Miescher S, Whiteside TL, Carrel S, Von Fliedner V. Functional properties of tumor-infiltrating and blood lymphocytes in patients with solid tumors: Effects of tumor

Table 2. Characteristics of TIL freshly recovered from human solid tumors

1.	Morphology:	small lymphocytes
2.	Phenotype:	$CD3^+TcR\text{-}\alpha/\beta^+$ T cells memory T cells ($CDw29^+$) frequently express activation antigens (CD25, HLA-DR) mixtures of $CD8^+$ and $CD4^+$
3.	Clonality:	oligoclonal in the TcR V β gene expression
4.	Function:	often depressed locomotion, proliferation, and antitumor cytotoxicity, as compared to autologous PBL. TIL may have a defect in the antigen-dependent activation pathway leading to proliferation
5.	In vitro response to IL-2:	many but not all TIL recover the ability to proliferate and lyse fresh tumor targets

cells and their supernatants on proliferative responses of lymphocytes. J Immunol 1986; 136:1899-1907.
7. Alexander JP, Kudoh S, Melsop KA, Hamilton TA, Edinger MG, Tubbs RR, Sica D, Tuason L, Klein E, Bukowski RM, Finke JH. T-cells infiltrating renal cell carcinoma display a poor proliferative response even though they can produce interleukin 2 and express interleukin 2 receptors. Cancer Res 1993; 53:1380-1387.
8. Moy PM, Holmes EC, Golub SH. Depression of natural killer cytotoxic activity in lymphocytes infiltrating human pulmonary tumors. Cancer Res 1985; 45:57-60.
9. Vose BM, Vanky F, Klein E. Human tumor-lymphocyte interaction in vitro. V. Comparison of the reactivity of tumor-infiltrating, blood and lymph-node lymphocytes with autologous tumor cells. Int J Cancer 1977; 20:895-902.
10. Hutchinson GH, Heinemann D, Symes MO, Williamson RCN. Differential immune reactivity of tumor-intrinsic and peripheral-blood lymphocytes against autoplastic colorectal carcinoma cells. Br J Cancer 1981; 44:396-402.
11. Klein E, Vanky F, Galili U, Vose BM, Fopp M. Separation and characterization of tumor-infiltrating lymphocytes in man. Contemp Top Immunol 1980; 10:79-107.
12. Totterman TH, Parthenais E, Hayry P, Timonen T, Saksela E. Cytological and functional analysis of inflammatory infiltrates in human malignant tumors. III. Further functional investigations using cultured autochthonous tumor cell lines and freeze-thawed infiltrating inflammatory cells. Cell Immunol 1980; 55:219-226.
13. Miescher S, Stoeck M, Whiteside TL, Leyvraz S, Ruzicka J, Schindler AM, Givel JC, Mosimann F, Von Fliedner V. Altered activation pathways in T lymphocytes infiltrating human solid tumors. Transplant Proc 1988; 20:344-346.
14. Miescher S, Stoeck M, Qiao L, Barras C, Barrelet L, Von Fliedner V. Proliferative and cytolytic potentials of purified human tumor-infiltrating T lymphocytes. Impaired response to mitogen-driven stimulation despite T-cell receptor expression. Int J Cancer 1988; 42:659-666.
15. Vose BM, Moore M. Suppressor cell activity of lymphocytes infiltrating human lung and breast tumors. Int J Cancer 1979; 24:579-585.
16. Chakraborty NG, Sporn JR, Pasquale DR, Ergin MT, Mukherji B. Suppression of lymphokine-activated killer cell generation by tumor-infiltrating lymphocytes. Clin Immunol Immunopathol 1991; 59:407-416.
17. Snyderman CH, Heo DS, Johnson JT, d'Amico F, Barnes L, Whiteside TL. Functional and phenotypic analysis of lymphocytes isolated from tumors and lymph nodes of patients with head and neck cancer. Arch Otolaryngol Head Neck Surg 1991; 117:899-905.
18. DeVries JE, Spits H. Cloned human cytotoxic T lymphocyte (CTL) lines reactive with autologous melanoma cells. I. In vitro generation, isolation and analysis of phenotype and specificity. J Immunol 1984; 132:510-519.
19. Mukherji B, MacAlister TJ. Clonal analysis of cytotoxic T-cell response against human melanoma. J Exp Med 1983; 158:240-245.
20. Vose BM, White W. Tumor-reactive lymphocytes stimulated in mixed lymphocyte and tumor culture. Clonal analysis of effector cells in cytotoxic and proliferative assays. Cancer Immunol Immunother 1983; 15:227-236.
21. Anichini A, Fossati G, Parmiani G. Clonal analysis of cytotoxic T-lymphocyte response to autologous human metastatic melanoma. Int J Cancer 1985; 35:683-689.
22. Uchida A, Klein E. Generation of cytotoxic factor by human large granular lymphocytes during interaction with autologous tumor cells: Lysis of fresh human tumor cells. JNCI 1988; 80:1398-1403.
23. Uchida A, Moore M, Klein E. Autologous mixed lymphocyte-tumor reaction and autologous mixed lymphocyte reaction. II. Generation of specific and non-specific killer T cells capable of lysing autologous tumor. Int J Cancer 1988; 41:651-656.
24. Miescher S, Stoeck M, Qiao L, Barras C, Barrelet L, Von Fliedner V. Preferential clonogenic deficit of CD8+ T lymphocytes infiltrating human solid tumors. Cancer Res

1988; 48:6992-6998.
25. Whiteside TL, Miescher S, Hurlimann J, Moretta L, Von Fliedner V. Clonal analysis and in situ characterization of lymphocytes infiltrating human breast carcinomas. Cancer Immunol Immunother 1986; 23:169-178.
26. Shimizu Y, Iwatsuki S, Herberman RB, Whiteside TL. Clonal analysis of tumor-infiltrating lymphocytes from human primary and metastatic liver tumors. Int J Cancer 1990; 46:878-883.
27. Biassoni R, Prigione I, Di Marco E, Ferrini S. Cytolytic activity of T lymphocytes isolated from ovarian carcinoma ascitic fluid. Analysis at the population and clonal level. La Ricerca Clin Lab 1985; 15:177-183.
28. Shimizu Y, Weidmann E, Iwatsuki S, Herberman RB, Whiteside TL. Characterization of human autotumor-reactive T-cell clones obtained from tumor-infiltrating lymphocytes in liver metastasis of gastric carcinoma. Cancer Res 1991; 51:6153-6162.
29. Applegate KG, Balch CM, Pellis NR. In vitro migration of lymphocytes through collagen matrix: arrested locomotion in tumor-infiltrating lymphocytes. Cancer Res 1990; 50:7153-7158.
30. Vitolo D, Letessier EM, Johnson JT, Whiteside TL. Immunologic effector cells in head and neck cancer. In: Biology of and Novel Therapeutic Approaches for Epithelial Cancers of the Aerodigestive Tract. JNCI Monographs, 1992: 203-208.
31. Schoof DD, Selleck CM, Massaro AF, Jung S-E, Eberlein TJ. Activation of human tumor-infiltrating lymphocytes by monoclonal antibodies directed to the CD3 complex. Cancer Res 1990; 50:1138-1143.
32. Zocchi MR, Poggi A, Crosti F, Tongiani S, Rugarli C. Signalling in human tumor-infiltrating lymphocytes: The CD28 molecule is functional and is physically associated with CD45RO molecule. Eur J Cancer 1992; 28A:749-754.
33. Shimizu Y, Iwatsuki S, Herberman RB, Whiteside TL. Effects of cytokines on in vitro growth of tumor-infiltrating lymphocytes obtained from human primary and metastatic liver tumors. Cancer Immunol Immunother 1991; 32:280-288.
34. Schwartz RH. A cell culture model for T lymphocyte clonal anergy. Science 1990; 248:1349-1356.
35. Pawelec G, Brocker T, Busch FW, Buhring HJ, Fernandez N, Schneider EM, Wernet P. "Tolerization" of human T-helper cell clones by chronic exposure to alloantigen: Culture conditions dictate autocrine proliferative status but not acquisition of cytotoxic potential and suppressor-induction capacity. J Mol Cell Immunol 1988; 4:21-34.
36. Snyderman R, Cianciolo GJ. Immunosuppressive activity of the retroviral envelope protein p15E and its possible relationship to neoplasia. Immunol Today 1984; 5:240-242.
37. Cianciolo GJ, Copeland TD, Oroszlan S, Snyderman R. Inhibition of lymphocyte proliferation by a synthetic peptide homologous to retroviral envelope proteins. Science 1985; 230:453-455.
38. Roth JA, Osborne BA, Ames RS. Immunoregulatory factors derived from human tumors. II. Partial purification and further immunobiochemical characterization of a human sarcoma-derived immunosuppressive factor expressing HLA-DR and immunoglobulin-related determinants. J Immunol 1983; 130:303-308.
39. Botha JH, Robinson KM, Ramchurren N, Reddi K, Norman RJ. Human esophageal carcinoma cell lines: Prostaglandin production, biological properties, and behavior in nude mice. JNCI 1986; 76:1053-1056.
40. Wrann M, Bodmer S, de Martin R, Siepl C, Hofer-Warbinek R, Frei K, Hofer E, Fontana A. T-cell suppressor factor from human glioblastoma cells is a 12.5 Kd protein closely related to transforming growth factor β. EMBO J 1987; 6:1633-1636.
41. Ebert EC, Roberts AI, O'Connell SM, Robertson FM, Nagase H. Characterization of an immunosuppressive factor derived from colon cancer cells. J Immunol 1987; 138:2161-2168.
42. Takagi S, Chen K, Schwarz R, Iwatsuki S, Herberman RB, Whiteside TL. Functional and phenotypic analysis of tumor-infiltrating lymphocytes isolated from human primary and metastatic liver tumors and cultured in recombinant interleukin 2. Cancer 1989; 63:102-111.
43. Heo DS, Whiteside TL, Kanbour A,

Herberman RB. Role of Leu19 (NKH1)-positive effector cells in mediating autologous and allogeneic tumor cell lysis in rIL-2-activated cultures of lymphocytes infiltrating human ovarian tumors. J Immunol 1988; 140:4042-4049.

44. Ioannides CG, Platsoucas CD, Rashed S, Wharton JT, Edwards CL, Freedman RS. Tumor cytolysis by lymphocytes infiltrating ovarian malignant ascites. Cancer Res 1991; 51:4257-4265.
45. Itoh K, Platsoucas CD, Balch CM. Autologous tumor-specific cytotoxic T lymphocytes in the infiltrate of human metastatic melanomas. Activation by interleukin 2 and autologous tumor cells, and involvement of the T-cell receptor. J Exp Med 1988; 168:1419-1441.
46. Yasumura S, Hirabayashi H, Schwartz DR, Toso JF, Johnson JT, Herberman RB, Whiteside TL. Human cytotoxic T-cell lines with restricted specificity for squamous cell carcinoma of the head and neck. Cancer Res 1993; 53:1461-1468.
47. Mukherji B, Guha A, Chakraborty NG, Sivanandham M, Nashed AL, Sporn JR, Ergin MT. Clonal analysis of cytotoxic and regulatory T-cell responses against human melanoma. J Exp Med 1989; 169:1961-1976.
48. Cozzolino F, Torcia M, Carossino AM, Giordani R, Selli C, Talini G, Reali E, Novelli A, Pistoia V, Ferrarini M. Characterization of cells from invaded lymph nodes in patients with solid tumors. J Exp Med 1987; 166:303-318.
49. Belldegrun A, Kasid A, Uppenkamp M, Topalian SL, Rosenberg SA. Human tumor-infiltrating lymphocytes: Analysis of lymphokine mRNA expression and relevance to cancer immunotherapy. J Immunol 1989; 42:4520-4526.
50. Erroi A, Sironi M, Chiaffarino F, Chen ZG, Mengozzi M, Mantovani A. IL-1 and IL-6 released by tumor-associated macrophages from human ovarian carcinoma. Int J Cancer 1989; 44:795-801.
51. Erroi A, Casali B, Donati MB, Mantovani A, Semeraro N. Mouse tumor-associated macrophages do not generate procoagulant activity in response to different stimuli. Int J Cancer 1988; 41:65-68.
52. Von Roenn J, Harris JE, Braun DP. Suppressor cell function in solid tumor cancer patients. J Clin Oncol 1987; 5:150-159.
53. Mukherji B, Chakraborty NG, Sivanandham MT. T-cell clones that react against autologous human tumors. Immunol Rev 1990; 116:33-62.
54. Letessier EM, Sacchi M, Johnson JT, Herberman RB, Whiteside TL. The absence of lymphoid suppressor cells in tumor-involved lymph nodes of patients with head and neck cancer. Cellular Immunol 1990; 130:446-458.
55. Weidmann E, Sacchi M, Plaisance S, Heo DS, Yasumura S, Lin WC, Johnson JT, Herberman RB, Azzarone B, Whiteside TL. Receptors for interleukin 2 on human squamous cell carcinoma cell lines and tumor in situ. Cancer Res 1992; 52:5963-5970.
56. Rimoldi D, Salvi S, Hartmann F, Schreyer M, Blum S, Zografos L, Plaisance S, Azzarone B, Carrel S. Expression of IL-2 receptors in human melanoma cells. AntiCancer Res 1993; 13:555-564.
57. Vitolo D, Zerbe T, Kanbour A, Dahl C, Herberman RB, Whiteside TL. Expression of mRNA for cytokines in tumor-infiltrating mononuclear cells in ovarian adenocarcinoma and invasive breast cancer. Int J Cancer 1992; 51:573-580.
58. Vitolo D, Kanbour A, Johnson JT, Herberman RB, Whiteside TL. In situ hybridization for cytokine gene transcripts in the solid tumor microenvironment. Eur J Cancer 1993; 3:371-377.
59. Ranges GE, Figari IS, Espevik T, Palladino MA,Jr. Inhibition of cytotoxic T-cell development by transforming growth factor β and reversal by recombinant tumor necrosis factor α. J Exp Med 1987; 166:991-998.
60. Tada T, Ohzeki S, Utsumi K, Takiuchi H, Muramatsu M, Li XF, Shimizu J, Fujiwara H, Hamaoka T. Transforming growth factor-β-induced inhibition of T-cell function. Susceptibility difference in T cells of various phenotypes and functions and its relevance to immunosuppression in the tumor-bearing state. J Immunol 1991; 146:1077-1082.
61. Yoshino I, Yano T, Yoshikai Y, Murata M, Sugimachi K, Kimura G, Nomoto K. Oligoclonal T lymphocytes infiltrating

human lung cancer tissues. Int J Cancer 1991; 47:654-658.
62. Lee HM, Rich S. Costimulation of T-cell proliferation by transforming growth factor-β 1. J Immunol 1991; 147:1127-1133.
63. Vaccarello L, Wang YL, Whiteside TL. Sustained outgrowth of autotumor-reactive T lymphocytes from human ovarian carcinomas in the presence of tumor necrosis factor α and interleukin 2. Human Immunol 1990; 28:216-227.
64. Wang YL, Si L, Kanbour A, Herberman RB, Whiteside TL. Lymphocytes infiltrating human ovarian tumors. Synergy between tumor necrosis factor α and interleukin 2 in the generation of CD8⁺ effectors from tumor-infiltrating lymphocytes. Cancer Res 1989; 49:5979-5985.
65. Ioannides CG, Rashed S, Fisk B, Fan D, Itoh K, Freedman RS. Lymphocytes infiltrating ovarian malignant ascites: modulation of IL-2-induced proliferation by IL-4 and of selective increase in CD8+ T cells by TNF-α. Lymphokine & Cytokine Res 1991; 10:307-315.
66. Takeyama H, Wakamiya N, O'Hara C, Arthur K, Niloff J, Kufe D, Sakarai K, Spriggs D. Tumor necrosis factor expression by human ovarian carcinoma in vivo. Cancer Res 1991; 51:4476-4480.
67. Radinsky T. Growth factors and their receptors in metastasis. Semin Cancer Biol 1991; 2:169-177.
68. Mead JE, Fausto N. Transforming growth factor α may be a physiological regulator of liver regeneration by means of an autocrine mechanism. PNAS USA 1989; 86:1558-1562.
69. Grupposo PA, Mead JE, Fausto N. Transforming growth factor receptors in liver regeneration following partial hepatectomy in the rat. Cancer Res 1990; 50:1464-1469.
70. Mizoguchi H, O'Shea JJ, Longo DL, Loeffler CM, McVicar DW, Ochoa AC. Alterations in signal transduction molecules in T lymphocytes from tumor-bearing mice. Science 1992; 258:1795-1798.
71. Loeffler CM, Smyth MJ, Longo DL, Kopp WC, Harvey LK, Tribble HR, Tase JE, Urba WJ, Leonard AS, Young HA, Ochoa AC. Immunoregulation in cancer-bearing hosts. Down-regulation of gene expression and cytotoxic function in CD8+ T cells. J Immunol 1992; 149:949-956.
72. Bodmer S, Strommer K, Frei K, Siepl C, deTribolet N, Heid I, Fontana A. Immunosuppression and transforming growth factor-β in glioblastoma. J Immunol 1989; 143:3222-3229.
73. Lopez DM, Lopez-Cepero M, Watson GA, Ganju A, Sotomayor E, Fu Y-X. Modulation of the immune system by mammary tumor-derived factors. Cancer Invest 1991; 9:643-653.
74. Packard BS. Mitogenic stimulation of human tumor-infiltrating lymphocytes by secreted factor(s) from human tumor cell lines. PNAS USA 1990; 87:4058-4062.
75. Rabinowich H, Vitolo D, Altarac S, Herberman RB, Whiteside TL. Role of cytokines in the adoptive immunotherapy of an experimental model of human head and neck cancer by human IL-2-activated natural killer cells. J Immunol 1992; 149:340-349.
76. Hirabayashi H, Yasumura S, Lin W-C, Amoscato A, Johnson JT, Herberman RB, Whiteside TL. Production by human squamous cell carcinomas of a factor inducing activation and proliferation of immune cells. Arch Otolaryngol Head Neck Surg 1993; In press.
77. Luger TA, Stadler BM, Luger BM, Sztein M, Schmidt JA, Hawley-Nelson P, Grabner G, Oppenheim JJ. Characteristic of an epidermal cell thymocyte-activating factor (ETAF) by human epidermal cells and a human squamous cell carcinoma cell line. J Invest Dermatol 1983; 81:187-93.
78. Luger TA, Charon JA, Colot M, Micksche M, Oppenheim JJ. Chemotactic properties of partially purified human epidermal cell-derived thymocyte-activating factor (ETAF) for polymorphonuclear and mononuclear cells. J Immunol 1983; 131:816-820.
79. Luger TA, Uchida A, Kock A, Colot M, Micksche M. Human epidermal cell and squamous carcinoma cells synthesize a cytokine that augments natural killer cell activity. J Immunol 1985; 134:2477-2483.

CHAPTER 6

In Vitro Expansion and Characteristics of Cultured TIL

While freshly isolated TIL are often unable to proliferate upon short-term (48–72h) exposure to IL-2, TIL cultured in the presence of IL-2 for several weeks acquire the ability to proliferate and to kill tumor cell targets.[1,2] Thus, IL-2 at relatively high concentrations (>100 Cetus U/ml or >600 IU/ml) appears to be the best and fairly "universal" agent for activating TIL and overcoming tumor-induced inhibition of proliferation. The potential for a reversal of TIL unresponsiveness in vitro has been explored using agents other than IL-2. For example, anti-CD3 or anti-TcR mAbs have been used to induce activation, proliferation, and effector function in freshly isolated or cultured human TIL, which do not respond to IL-2 alone.[3-7] Studies in other systems have shown that while anti-CD3 mAb can induce unresponsiveness in unprimed T cells, previously primed T cells such as TIL are responsive to anti-CD3 mAb.[8] Cytokines other than IL-2, e.g., IL-4, or combinations of cytokines have also been tried with various degrees of success to induce or augment in vitro activation and proliferation of TIL obtained from human tumors.[9-11] In fact, recombinant cytokines have been universally employed to generate large numbers of TIL required for immunotherapy of human tumors.

In this chapter, phenotypic and functional characteristics of TIL cultured in the presence of cytokines will be reviewed. Evidence has accumulated that it is possible to generate AuTu-specific CTL from TIL. Attributes of tumor-specific CTL thus generated, and the practicality of using CTL-derived from TIL for immune therapy of cancer will be discussed, because of an increasing interest in generation of well-characterized and highly active antitumor effector cells. Culture conditions which might facilitate reproducible outgrowth of CTL from TIL or reduce proportions of nontumor specific LAK cells will be evaluated as will the ability of tumor cells to sustain in vitro immune response to the tumor. Cultured TIL represent a source of antitumor effector cells, but a controversy has developed as to whether TIL are the best and preferable source of such effector cells, given the difficulty and considerable expense associated with TIL isolation and expansion. To solve this controversy, it appears reasonable to compare TIL with other known effector cells used for therapy, such as LAK or purified human NK cells, and make a rational decision about their antitumor potential. The aim of this chapter is to review the data available on properties of cultured TIL and to aid the reader in formulating an objective and informed view of TIL as an appropriate source of therapeutically-promising effector cells.

EXPANSION OF TIL IN THE PRESENCE OF IL-2

The presence of exogenous IL-2 is required for proliferation of human TIL in culture. However, even if TIL are cultured in a high concentration of IL-2, they do not always respond by proliferation as extensive as that described for TIL from human melanomas.[2,12] For example, among 44 TIL preparations obtained in our laboratory from primary human solid tumors other than melanomas, 7 did not proliferate in the presence of IL-2, while autologous PBL proliferated as expected.[2,13] Similarly, in patients with head and neck cancer, some TIL preparations did not proliferate, although median expansion for TIL in long-term cultures was higher than that for A-PBL (Fig. 1). TIL obtained from colon carcinomas metastatic to liver had different kinetics and magnitude of expansion in response to IL-2 than those from primary liver tumors (see Fig. 2).[12,14] The former frequently proliferated only after a lag of several days and following expansion, had significantly lower antitumor cytotoxicity in bulk cultures.[12,14] In general, TIL from primary solid tumors proliferated better than A-PBL in the presence of IL-2. However, on a per cell basis, these TIL and PBL in culture had comparable antitumor cytotoxicity when tested in 4h ^{51}Cr-release assays against autologous or allogeneic tumor cell targets.[2,15] Due to better growth of TIL, total lytic units of antitumor cytotoxicity were often higher for TIL than A-PBL for a variety of cancers such as RCC, melanomas, SCCHN, ovarian or colon carcinomas.[2,15-18]

While TIL obtained from metastatic disease were significantly less responsive to IL-2 in bulk cultures than those from primary cancers,[12] the major issue has been the nature of cytotoxic antitumor effector cells generated in these cultures. Two-color flow cytometry analyses showed that TIL cultured in IL-2 were as heterogeneous as LAK-cell cultures established from PBL, comprising CD3$^+$CD56$^-$, CD3$^+$CD56$^+$ and CD3$^-$CD56$^+$ cell subsets in various

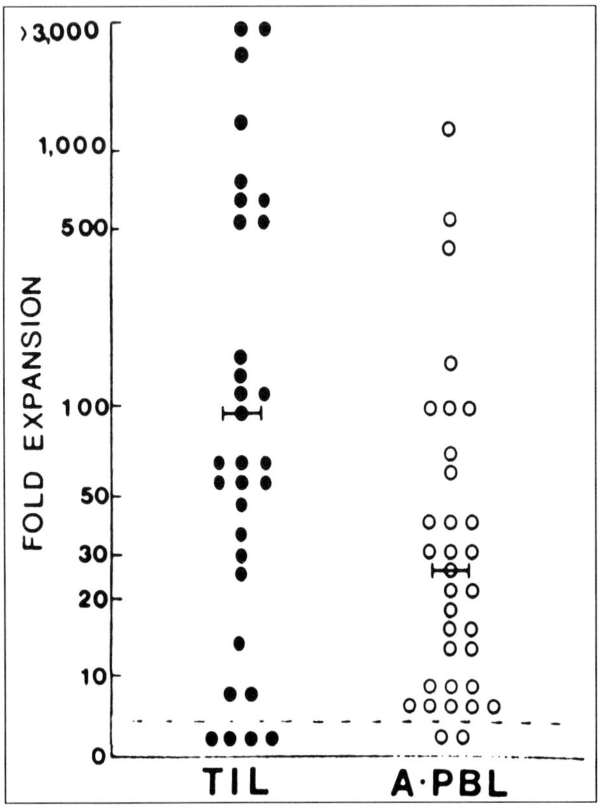

Fig. 1. Expansion achieved in long-term cultures in the presence of IL-2 (6000 IU/ml) by tumor-infiltrating lymphocytes (TIL) and autologous peripheral blood lymphocytes (A-PBL) obtained from patients with head and neck tumors. The median expansion for each group is designated by the bar. The interrupted line separates those cultures that did not expand under the experimental conditions used. Reproduced with permission from Whiteside et al, Cancer Immunol Immunother 1988;26:1-10.

proportions.[13,16,18] The ratios of CD4⁺/CD8⁺ T cells were equally variable in these cultures, with the only exception of TIL from melanomas which often, but certainly not always, outgrew more homogeneous populations of CD3⁺CD8⁺ effectors with AuTu cytotoxicity.[1,19,20] In a great majority of TIL preparations grown in the presence of IL-2 by us and others, effector cells generated in bulk cultures were phenotypically and functionally similar to autologous LAK cells in the peripheral blood.[17,18,21,22] The anticipated enrichment in AuTu-specific CD3⁺CD8⁺ effector cells was difficult to achieve in TIL cultures, even after an initial enrichment in CD8⁺ T cells by, e.g., negative selection on mAb-coated flasks and expansion in IL-2.[23,24]

EXPANSION OF TIL IN THE PRESENCE OF COMBINED CYTOKINES

To improve the feasibility of outgrowing CD3⁺ CD8⁺ class I MHC-restricted effector cells rather than CD3⁻CD56⁺ NK cells or CD3⁺CD56⁺ non-MHC-restricted T cells from TIL preparations, mixtures of IL-2 with other cytokines have been employed.[9-11,25-29] The rationale for this approach came from studies with murine TIL, which showed that additions at optimal concentrations of IFN-γ, TNF-α, IL-4 or IL-7[10,11,30-32] to culture media containing IL-2 enhanced the development of cytotoxic T cells. Synergistic antitumor interactions of IL-2, IFN-α and TIL have been described in mice and led to a concept of combination immunotherapy for cancer.[33] Based on these studies in animal models, combinations of various cytokines, e.g., IL-2 and TNF-α[26,27] or IL-2 and IL-4[9,34] have been recently used to obtain TIL cultures enriched in AuTu-reactive T lymphocytes in patients with solid tumors. For example, in our hands, the combination of IL-2 (100 U/ml) and TNF-α (1,000 U/ml) was quite effective in promoting enrichment of autotumor-reactive CD3⁺CD8⁺ T lymphocytes in long-term cultures of TIL obtained from human ovarian carcinomas[26,29] or primary liver tumors.[14] IL-2 alone induced growth of effectors with non-MHC-restricted cytotoxicity.[14] Additions

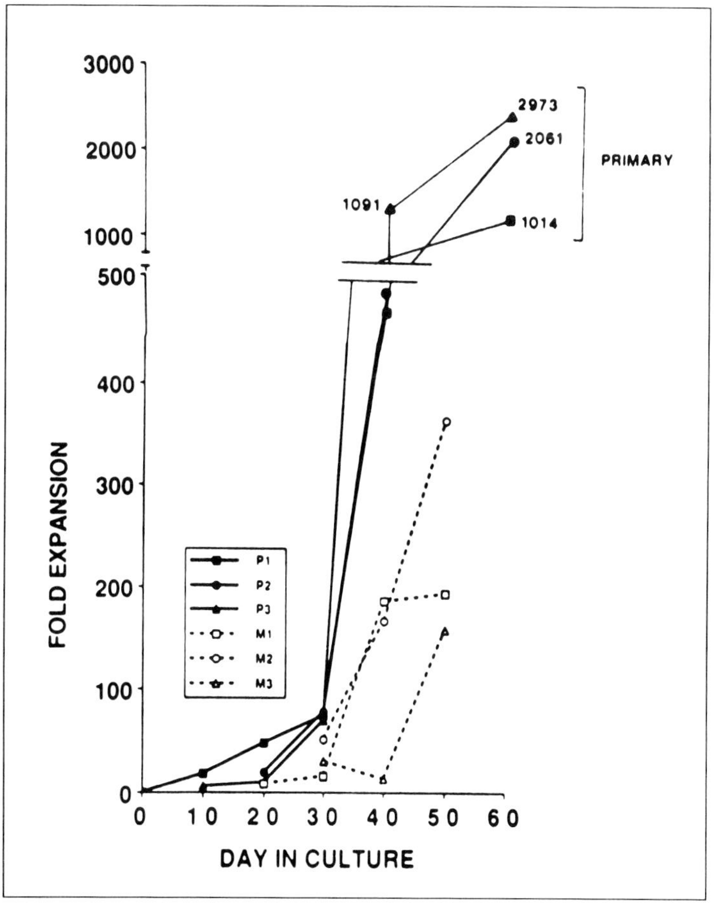

Fig. 2. Kinetics of expansion in cultures in the presence of IL-2 (6000 IU/ml) of TIL obtained from three patients with hepatocellular carcinoma and three patients with colon carcinoma metastasized to the liver. The numbers indicate the final fold expansion of TIL obtained from primary liver tumors. Note that TIL obtained from liver metastases and cultured under the same conditions were delayed in growth and did not the achieve fold proliferation comparable to that of TIL from primary liver tumors. Reproduced with permission from Takagi et al, Cancer 1989;63:102-111.

of IFN-γ or IL-4 to these TIL cultures did not result in improved selected growth of autotumor-reactive $CD3^+CD8^+$ T cells. In agreement with generally poorer growth of TIL from metastatic than primary tumors referred to earlier, TIL from colon adenocarcinomas metastatic to liver showed both limited expansion and less cytotoxicity against AuTu cells regardless of which cytokine or cytokine combinations were used in culture.[14] The precise mechanism involved in preferential outgrowth of $CD3^+CD8^+$ T lymphocytes from TIL in the presence of IL-2 and TNF-α or other cytokines is not understood. It has been proposed that TNF-α might reverse inhibition of CTL induced in vivo by tumor-derived TGF-β.[35] An alternative explanation might be that TNF-α increases immunogenicity of a tumor by e.g., up-regulating the expression of class I MHC Ags on its surface.[36] Not all combinations of cytokines are equally effective for TIL from different tumors. In melanoma, IL-2 and IL-4 were reported to augment the growth and cytotoxicity of TIL specific for AuTu,[34] but the same combination of cytokines did not have augmenting effects in cultures of TIL from primary liver tumors.[14] Nevertheless, certain cytokine combinations promote outgrowth of $CD8^+$ populations of T lymphocytes with restricted specificity from TIL obtained from a variety of human solid tumors,[29] and this seems to indicate that AuTu-specific $CD8^+$ T lymphocytes are a component of these TIL in situ.

OUTGROWTH OF AUTU-SPECIFIC CTL FROM TIL

The above considerations focus attention on culture conditions which might determine selective and reproducible outgrowth from TIL of CTL or reduce proportions of tumor non-specific LAK cells. Among variables that could considerably influence selective outgrowth of AuTu-specific T cells are the presence of irradiated AuTu cells, additions of APC and feeder cells, and the concentration of IL-2. At the same time, establishing what may be optimal culture conditions for TIL from one solid tumor (e.g., 5-50 U/ml of IL-2 in the presence of 10 to 100 lymphocytes per tumor cell and of autologous lymphoblastoid B-cell line as APC) does not guarantee that TIL from another tumor, even of the same histologic type, will respond in the same way. In fact, the presence of AuTu in such cultures may be inhibitory, if the tumor produces immunoinhibitory factors such as TGF-β or PGE_2.[37,38] In such cases, as for example with those SCCHN which produce copious amounts of PGE_2,[39] cell membrane fractions rather than whole tumor cells or synthetic peptides might be a more suitable immunostimulatory signal for TIL in culture. Overall, many variables determine the outcome of TIL cultures, and optimal conditions for selection of CTL in vitro may have to be tailored to individual TIL preparations.

Perhaps the most critical single parameter which determines the presence of CTL in the tumor is its immunogenicity or ability to evoke and sustain the host immune response specifically directed at the tumor. That is, human tumors which express immunogenic TAA in the context of class I MHC Ags and present these Ags effectively to the immune system are expected to be well infiltrated with CTL. Such appears to be the case in human melanomas, where both the existence of CTL in the circulation[40,41] as well as in cultured TIL[19,20,42] and of melanoma Ags capable of evoking development of CTL in vitro[43] have been clearly documented. In melanoma, class I MHC molecules are well expressed in most of the primary and metastatic lesions.[44,45] Guerry and his collaborators showed that melanoma cells effectively process Ag, present it to T cells, and secrete IL-1,[46] leaving little doubt that melanomas, especially in early disease stages, are immunogenic. Although CTL with specificity for AuTu have been obtained from peripheral blood or TIL of some patients with cancer, in most patients, it has not been possible to document the presence of such T cells in the periphery or at the tumor site. Recently, we have reported generation and characterization of CTL with specificity restricted to AuTu and a small number of allogeneic SCCHN from peripheral blood of a patient with SCC of the tongue.[47] While all attempts at establishing a CTL line from this patient's PBL over a period of over two years have been successful, we have failed to establish CTL from PBL or TIL of ten other individuals with SCCHN for whom AuTu cell lines and cryopreserved CTL were available, utilizing the same experimental conditions.[47] Even in patients with melanoma, anti-melanoma-specific responses develop in vitro in only 30-50% of cases using lymph node lymphocytes, PBL or TIL as sources of effector cells.[48] In other solid tumors, generation of AuTu-specific responses seems to occur even less frequently,[49] and it has not been confirmed that human TIL are consistently a better source of CTL than are circulating T lymphocytes.

Considerable efforts have been made in the last few years to define in vitro conditions for generation and expansion of AuTu-specific CTL from TIL obtained from various human tumors. In several studies, greater cell yields as well as increased and prolonged cytotoxic activity of TIL against AuTu were achieved by utilizing multiple restimulations of TIL cultured in the presence of low or moderate doses of IL-2 with AuTu.[50-52] However, restimulation in vitro with AuTu did not consistently result in the generation of specific CTL from TIL. The goal of outgrowing AuTu-specific TIL with consistency has not been achieved so far even with melanoma TIL. While restimulation of TIL with AuTu may be beneficial, it is both difficult to implement because of a requirement for a substantial number of AuTu cells and by no means as reliable as expected.

The nature of antigenic determinants recognized by AuTu-specific CTL is largely unknown and a subject of intense investigation at present. In general, AuTu-specific CTL express the $CD3^+CD8^+TcR\text{-}\alpha/\beta^+$ phenotype and ability to kill AuTu targets as a result of class I MHC-restricted Ag recognition on these targets.[53-58] In mice, melanomas which lacked expression of class I MHC Ags were not immunogenic, and TIL obtained from these tumors had no AuTu cytotoxicity.[59] But TIL recovered from the same tumors transfected with the class I MHC gene specifically lysed AuTu and caused tumor regression.[59] Thus, tumor immunogenicity, association of tumor Ag with class I MHC Ags on the tumor cell surface and processing of TAA by APC are required for development of CTL in patients with solid tumors. It has been suggested that a class I MHC molecule-peptide complex on the surface of tumor cells is recognized by the tumor-specific CTL via the TcR.[60] More precisely, it appears that epitopes recognized by the T cell are presented as antigenic peptides eight to ten amino acids in length, which contain a binding or anchor site for the HLA molecule (4-5 amino acids) and a second binding site for the TcR.[60,61] Both shared/common and unique TAA recognized by CTL and restricted by HLA-A1 or HLA-A2 elements have been reported for human melanoma.[57,58,62,63]

Not all tumor-specific CTL are class I restricted, however. T lymphocyte lines established from lymph nodes draining pancreatic carcinomas, which were $CD3^+$ $CD8^+TcR\text{-}\alpha/\beta^+$ and recognized pancreatic carcinoma-associated mucins, were independent of the MHC in recognition of the target Ag. Antibodies to class I or class II MHC Ags did not interfere with cytolytic functions of these T cells, while anti-CD3 mAbs abolished cytotoxicity.[64,65] Thus, some TAA, specifically, large, polyvalent and heavily glycosylated mucins associated with pancreatic or breast tumors, appear to be able to activate mucin-specific CTL directly without a need for Ag presentation or processing.[66,67] More recent studies of Finn and her collaborators indicate that mucin-specific CTL may be quite common in lymph nodes or peripheral blood of patients with pancreatic, breast or ovarian cancer, because their isolation and culture are easily accomplished in most patients.[66,67] These mucin-specific T cells have been shown to recognize core mucin peptides, accessible to CTL, because mucins expressed on tumors are under-glycosylated in comparison to mucins expressed on normal epithelial cells.[66] Studies are ongoing in several laboratories aimed at the definition of various tumor-associated peptides and constructing synthetic peptide analogs which might be instrumental in improving our understanding of immunologically active versus silent TAA.

CLONAL ANALYSIS OF CTL OBTAINED FROM TIL

The clonal analyses of TIL have been performed in several laboratories in recent years, and they have resulted in several important conclusions regarding the nature of local CTL responses in human tumors. First, frequencies of CTL-p appear to be higher in TIL than A-PBL.[68] This has been observed in spite of lower PTL-p frequency of most TIL, as described earlier, with a preferential proliferation of $CD4^+$ and not $CD8^+$ T lymphocytes under culture conditions commonly used for LDA.[69,70] Second, although most of CTL-p in TIL give rise to cytolytic T-cell clones which are non-MHC-restricted,[69] TIL obtained from various tumors have been found to contain a variable proportion of T-cell clones restricted in cytotoxicity to AuTu. In TIL obtained from human primary liver tumors and recently cloned by LDA in our laboratory, the frequency of CTL-p for AuTu was 0.02-0.13, and 12/81 clones obtained were selectively reactive against AuTu.[68] Also, CTL-p for AuTu were not detected among cells from fresh A-PBL in these patients. Anichini and colleagues report that in melanoma, at least one melanoma-specific $CD3^+CD8^+$ TcR α/β^+ CTL clone can be found among 15 TIL clones screened for specificity using a panel of allogeneic melanomas including AuTu.[71] Third, the frequency of CTL clones with AuTu specificity appears to be lower in TIL from metastatic than primary tumors,[68] but even from TIL of a gastric carcinoma metastatic to liver, it was possible to establish recently three AuTu specific cytolytic clones which were $CD3^+$ $CD8^+$TcR $\alpha/\beta^+\gamma/\delta^-$, interacted with AuTu via the TcR, were class I MHC-restricted in killing of AuTu and selectively proliferated in response to AuTu.[55] Another important finding has been that TIL clones, even those expressing antitumor cytotoxicity, are frequently $CD4^+$, even in melanoma.[72] Some of $CD4^+$ clones obtained by us from TIL in hepatic tumors lysed AuTu but not K562, Daudi or allogeneic tumor cells.[68] Parmiani's group generated $CD4^+$ clones from melanoma TIL which were not cytotoxic to AuTu but which proliferated (and presumably secreted cytokines) selectively in response to AuTu.[72] Finally, clones of TIL-T seem to be very different from each other, even within the same TIL preparations, in terms of phenotype, cytokine profile, specificity for TAA and functions they can mediate.[48] In an elegant study, Mukherji and colleagues obtained both $CD4^+$ and $CD8^+$ T-cell lines from TIL or LNL of patients with melanoma and cultured them in the presence of AuTu and IL-2. In their hands, the $CD4^+$ lines established displayed either suppressive or helper functions independent their phenotype.[73]

In our recent study of over 200 clones obtained from the peripheral blood of a patient with SCCHN, six $CD8^+$ AuTu-specific cytotoxic clones were obtained, three of which expressed V β-6 and were restricted to killing SCCHN expressing HLA-A2 and the other three expressed V β-2 and were HLA-B44 restricted.[74] These CTL clones had the following functional properties: (a) the CTL-mediated lysis of AuTu was equally inhibited by mAbs to CD3, CD8, TcR-α/β or class I MHC Ag; (b) V β-6^+ clones represented a major proportion of the CTL line at ten weeks of culture, when AuTu cytotoxicity was at its peak. Later in culture, V β-2^+ T-cell clones which also mediated AuTu cytotoxicity, became a predominant cultured CTL population; (c) CTL clones incubated in the presence of AuTu (HLA-$A2^+$, $B44^+$) or HLA-matched allogeneic SCCHN targets, but not in the presence of unrelated HLA-$A2^+$ gastric carcinoma cells, produced cytokines TNF-α, IFN-γ and GM-CSF. An antigenic epitope(s) recognized on SCCHN targets by these CTL clones was apparently restricted by class I MHC antigens A2 or B44.[74] The observation that lysis by CTL of AuTu and HLA-matched allogeneic tumors can be inhibited with antibodies directed against class I MHC molecules or against the TcR, indicated that CTL recognized TAA in the context of class I MHC determinants. This study also suggested that more than one clonally-restricted AuTu-specific population of T cells could be generated from the peripheral blood of a patient with SCCHN in response to simulation with AuTu.[74]

It was initially believed that the putative

human tumor Ags were restricted to individual tumors. Recently, it has become apparent that the MHC-restricted recognition of allogeneic targets may occur if tumor targets share the class I MHC determinants with the effector cells. These findings suggest the presence of common or shared Ags on the tumors which may be recognized by the T cell.[42,56,75] Although the nature of these Ags remains largely unknown, the presence of both private and common tumor Ag has been inferred from the evidence that the same effector cells which lyse a group of allogeneic tumors in an MHC-restricted, and often HLA-A2-associated fashion, fail to lyse other tumor targets which share the same presenting element. Such resistant tumor targets are sensitive to lysis by autologous CTL. As recently reported by Boon's group, melanoma-associated antigens belonging to the MAGE family are likely candidates for common or shared tumor Ags recognized by HLA-A1$^+$ effector cells.[43,53,58]

CYTOKINE PRODUCTION BY CULTURED TIL

Human TIL obtained from patients with RCC or melanoma and cultured in the presence of exogenous IL-2 have been shown to express mRNA for various cytokines, including GM-CSF, TNF-α, TNF-β and IFN-γ[76] and to produce small amounts of these cytokines.[77] However, when cultured TIL were stimulated with AuTu, production of cytokines was specifically and significantly upregulated. Some TIL grown from human breast carcinomas or melanomas were shown to release GM-CSF, IFN-γ and TNF-α specifically in response to AuTu but not to a limited panel of allogeneic tumors or Epstein-Barr virus (EBV)-transformed B-cell lines.[77] Studies of TIL obtained from two melanoma patients and separated into CD4$^+$ and CD8$^+$ populations showed that CD8$^+$ cells were responsible for virtually all of the cytokine secretion, although both populations were able to release cytokines when activated by immunobilized anti-CD3 mAb.[77] In melanoma, AuTu-induced cytokine release by CD8$^+$ TIL was inhibited by anti-class I MHC mAb. In one case of TIL obtained from a patient with breast cancer, cytokine production by CD4$^+$ cells in response to fresh AuTu was inhibited by the anti-class II MHC mAb.[77]

The ability of AuTu-reactive T cells to release cytokines in the presence of AuTu cells is considered to be an indicator of specific recognition by TIL of TAA expressed by the tumor. It was initially believed that this role was reserved for tumor-specific, or perhaps autoreactive, CD4$^+$ T cells. Lymphokines usually released by helper CD4$^+$ T cells, IL-2, TNF-α, IFN-γ and IL-4, were thought to be essential for functional activation of CD8$^+$ cytolytic effector T cells.[78] The recent observation that human CD8$^+$ T cells can also secrete lymphokines, although at somewhat lower levels than CD4$^+$ cells,[79] and that CD8$^+$ TIL maintained in culture with IL-2 are specifically induced to secrete lymphokines in response to AuTu indicate that CD8$^+$ lymphocytes sensitized in vitro are good producers of cytokines.[77] In a study designed to determine if recognition of shared melanoma Ag can also induce cytokine release, Hom et al[80] co-cultured seven melanoma TIL, which lysed AuTu, with AuTu or with 7-12 HLA-matched or unmatched melanoma stimulators for 6-24h. SNs were collected and assayed by ELISA for the presence of GM-CSF, IFN-γ, TNF-α, IL-4, and IL6. Among five of six melanoma TIL for which AuTu was available, autologous melanoma cells stimulated specific release of at least one of three cytokines: GM-CSF, IFN-γ and TNF-α. Neither IL-4 nor IL-6 secretion by three TIL cultures tested was enhanced upon contact with tumor. For six of seven TIL cultures, HLA-matched allogeneic melanomas also stimulated significant cytokine release; HLA-A1, -A2, -A24, -B8 and -Cw7 were identified as possible restriction elements. The cytokine secretion induced by both autologous and allogeneic HLA-matched melanomas could be blocked by an anti-MHC I antibody.[80] These data suggested that cytokines could be specifically released by TIL recognizing a shared melanoma antigen in the context of self-MHC molecules.[80] In addition, in five of seven TIL studied, cytokine secretion correlated with cytolytic activity:

only tumors lysed by TIL stimulated specific cytokine release. However, for some TIL, tumor lysis and stimulation did not correlate. Thus, Hom et al suggest that these two TIL functions, cytotoxicity and cytokine production, represent separate mechanisms by which T cells can specifically interact with tumor. On the other hand, in TIL cultures established from patients with RCC and studied by Koo et al,[51] the degree of TNF-α mRNA expression appeared to correlate with the degree of AuTu-specific cytotoxicity of these TIL. Also, it is still unproven that tumors other than melanoma or RCC can specifically induce cytokine production by either fresh or IL-2-activated cultured TIL.

The ability of TIL to produce a range of cytokines following AuTu stimulation has received significant attention recently upon the demonstration in an experimental tumor model that the therapeutic potential of murine TIL correlated better with specific release of TNF-α and IFN-γ than with antitumor cytotoxicity, as measured in vitro.[81,82] Currently, studies are in progress to establish the correlation of specific cytokine release with therapeutic efficacy of TIL cultured for therapy. If such a correlation could be established, it would provide an important and useful in vitro correlate of TIL efficacy.

COMPARISON OF TIL, LAK AND NK CELLS AS ANTITUMOR EFFECTOR CELLS

Cellular antitumor immune responses in man appear to be heterogeneous in that both in vivo and in vitro a wide spectrum of antitumor-reactive effector cells may be elicited. These may include: TcR- and MHC-restricted AuTu-specific CTL;[43] TcR-restricted but MHC-unrestricted CTL, similar to T cells generated in response to tumor-associated mucins;[64,66] TcR- and MHC-unrestricted LAK cells as well as populations of activated NK cells.[83] Cultures of TIL in the presence of cytokines consist of heterogeneous mixtures of effector cells, which might include all or only some of the effectors listed above.[84] It is likely that the tumor microenvironment and other factors such as the nature and presentation of the TAA, ability of the tumor to produce chemotactic,[85] immunosuppressive,[86] or even immunostimulatory[87] factors, the presence of suppressor-regulatory cells, and local production of cytokines may all determine the nature of local cellular immune response against the tumor and also in vitro responses of TIL to cytokines. Although the presence in TIL cultures of AuTu-specific CTL has been largely confirmed, their recognition and selective expansion has been difficult to achieve, mainly because of the lack or paucity of AuTu cells for sensitization of effector cells in vitro and of AuTu as well as allogeneic tumor targets for cytotoxicity assays. Cytokine-activated NK cells and T cells are able to lyse NK-resistant targets, including AuTu.[88,89] Such "promiscuous", IL-2-induced behavior of TIL in culture makes it obligatory to resort to cloning by limiting dilution and clonal analyses in order to identify specific cytolytic or helper T cells among TIL from solid tumors.[90]

Fresh human TIL contain few NK cells,[91-93] and TIL expanding in vitro are rarely enriched in $CD3^-CD56^+$ effector cells. Rather, TIL in long-term cultures represent mixtures of $CD3^+CD56^+$ and $CD3^+CD56^-$ T cells which, to a large extent, are not AuTu specific or MHC-restricted and are, in fact, polyclonal with respect to the TcR V β gene expression.[94] Furthermore, clonal composition and expression of the V β or V α genes in TIL cultures changes over time, with AuTu-reactive clones generally outgrowing early, i.e., by week two to three in culture, and other clones, without AuTu-reactivity, gaining prominence in late TIL cultures.[94]

SUMMARY

Functional studies and RT-PCR performed with fresh and cultured TIL to determine their TcR V α and V β repertoire suggest that TIL are mixtures of polyclonal CTL, each recognizing a different antigenic epitope via the specific V β chain of the TcR or mixtures of polyclonal CTL restricted in their usage of V β chain genes or, alternatively, clonal proliferations of V β chain-restricted CTL recognizing one common or limited number of tumor Ags. The in situ PCR analysis of V α or V β gene usage by TIL indicates that the second or third alternatives might apply to TIL in ocular melanoma,[95] but the V β chain repertoire of fresh TIL has been examined in only a few other human tumors, and conclusions regarding the V β or α chain usage by TIL must await further studies. If fresh TIL prove to have a restricted TcR repertoire, it is possible that TIL expanding in vitro as clones or lines activated by exogenous cytokines might to a certain extent retain this restriction and represent a source enriched in cytolytic effector cells, at least some of which see or recognize a specific epitope on AuTu. At least in melanoma, such CTL have been selected from TIL maintained in culture and used as probes for TAA.[43,95-97]

The search for CTL among TIL from human solid tumors has been largely based on murine experiments which convincingly demonstrated that CTL can be generated from tumors[98] or lymphoid organs of tumor bearing animals.[99] That CTL also exist in most human tumors appears now pretty certain. However, a possibility that these CTL are inactive or immunosuppressed in vivo should be considered. Certainly, the hypothesis that TIL are a better source of AuTu-specific CTL than PBL or LNL has not been proven. It remains uncertain whether attempts to activate and grow CTL in vitro in the presence of cytokines are successful in selected instances only, and the optimal conditions for their culture have not yet been defined. From a therapeutic point of view the use of AuTu-specific effector cells may be advantageous, as discussed below; nevertheless, specific AIT with clonally-restricted TIL makes sense only if these effector cells recognize an epitope present on most AuTu cells. Given a well-known heterogeneity of human solid tumors, it seems unlikely that a single CTL clone will be therapeutically effective. On the other hand, if TIL can be manipulated in vitro in such a way as to expand into several AuTu specific clones, their therapeutic potential may indeed be important.

At present, no reliable in vitro correlate of therapeutic efficacy of TIL has been identified. Recent observations which indicate that cultured TIL can be specifically induced by AuTu to release certain cytokines and that this ability of TIL may correlate with their antitumor cytotoxicity and particularly with their therapeutic efficacy deserves further study. It seems to be essential to identify and evaluate an in vitro correlate of TIL clinical efficacy in the near future in order to be able to estimate with reasonable accuracy the therapeutic potential of TIL preparations and offer practical guidelines for TIL generation and therapy.

References

1. Itoh K, Tilden AB, Balch CM. Interleukin 2 activation of cytotoxic T lymphocytes infiltrating into human metastatic melanomas. Cancer Res 1986; 46:3011-3017.
2. Heo DS, Whiteside TL, Johnson JT, Chen K, Barnes EL, Herberman RB. Long-term interleukin 2-dependent growth and cytotoxic activity of tumor-infiltrating lymphocytes (TIL) from human squamous cell carcinomas of the head and neck. Cancer Res 1987; 47:6353-6362.
3. Miescher S, Stoeck M, Whiteside TL, Leyvraz S, Ruzicka J, Schindler AM, Givel JC, Mosimann F, Von Fliedner V. Altered activation pathways in T lymphocytes infiltrating human solid tumors. Transplant Proc 1988; 20:344-346.
4. Miescher S, Stoeck M, Qiao L, Barras C, Barrelet L, Von Fliedner V. Proliferative and cytolytic potentials of purified human tumor-infiltrating T lymphocytes. Impaired response to mitogen-driven stimulation despite T-cell receptor expression. Int J Cancer 1988; 42:659-666.
5. Alexander JP, Kudoh S, Melsop KA, Hamilton TA, Edinger MG, Tubbs RR, Sica D, Tuason L, Klein E, Bukowski RM, Finke JH. T-cells infiltrating renal cell carcinoma display a poor proliferative response even though they can produce interleukin 2 and express interleukin 2 receptors. Cancer Res 1993; 53:1380-1387.
6. Schoof DD, Jung SE, Eberlein TJ. Human tumor-infiltrating lymphocytes (TIL) cytotoxicity facilitated by anti-T-cell receptor antibody. Int J Cancer 1989; 44:219-224.
7. Schoof DD, Selleck CM, Massaro AF, Jung S-E, Eberlein TJ. Activation of human tumor-infiltrating lymphocytes by monoclonal antibodies directed to the CD3 complex.

Cancer Res 1990; 50:1138-1143.
8. Anasetti C, Tan P, Hansen JA, Martin PJ. Induction of specific nonresponsiveness in unprimed human T cells by anti-CD3 antibody and alloantigen. J Exp Med 1990; 172:1691-1700.
9. Kawakami Y, Custer MC, Rosenberg SA, Lotze MT. IL-4 regulates IL-2 induction of lymphokine-activated killer activity from human lymphocytes. J Immunol 1989; 142:3452-3461.
10. Stotter H, Custer MC, Bolton ES, Guedez L, Lotze MT. IL-7 induces human lymphokine-activated killer cell activity and is regulated by IL-4. J Immunol 1991; 146:150-155.
11. Stotter H, Lotze MT. Cytolytic effector cells against human tumors: Distinguishing phenotype and function. Cancer Cells 1990; 2:44-46-51-5.
12. Takagi S, Chen K, Schwarz R, Iwatsuki S, Herberman RB, Whiteside TL. Functional and phenotypic analysis of tumor-infiltrating lymphocytes isolated from human primary and metastatic liver tumors and cultured in recombinant interleukin 2. Cancer 1989; 63:102-111.
13. Whiteside TL, Heo DS, Takagi S, Johnson JT, Iwatsuki S, Herberman RB. Cytotoxic antitumor effector cells in long-term cultures of human tumor-infiltrating lymphocytes in recombinant IL-2. Cancer Immunol Immunother 1988; 26:1-10.
14. Shimizu Y, Iwatsuki S, Herberman RB, Whiteside TL. Effects of cytokines on in vitro growth of tumor-infiltrating lymphocytes obtained from human primary and metastatic liver tumors. Cancer Immunol Immunother 1991; 32:280-288.
15. Yoo YK, Heo DS, Hata K, Van Thiel DH, Whiteside TL. Tumor-infiltrating lymphocytes from human colon carcinomas. Functional and phenotypic characteristics after long-term culture in recombinant interleukin 2. Gastroenterol 1990; 98:259-268.
16. Heo DS, Whiteside TL, Kanbour A, Herberman RB. Role of Leu19 (NKH1)-positive effector cells in mediating autologous and allogeneic tumor cell lysis in rIL-2-activated cultures of lymphocytes infiltrating human ovarian tumors. J Immunol 1988; 140:4042-4049.
17. Belldegrun A, Muul LN, Rosenberg SA. Interleukin 2-expanded tumor-infiltrating lymphocytes in human renal cell cancer: Isolation, characterization, and antitumor activity. Cancer Res 1988; 48:206-214.
18. Whiteside TL, Heo DS, Takagi S, Herberman RB. Characterization of novel antitumor effector cells in long-term cultures of human tumor-infiltrating lymphocytes. Transpl Proc 1988; 20:347-350.
19. Muul LM, Spiess PJ, Director EP, Rosenberg SA. Identification of specific cytolytic immune responses against autologous tumor in humans bearing malignant melanoma. J Immunol 1987; 138:989-995.
20. Itoh K, Platsoucas CD, Balch CM. Autologous tumor-specific cytotoxic T lymphocytes in the infiltrate of human metastatic melanomas. Activation by interleukin 2 and autologous tumor cells, and involvement of the T-cell receptor. J Exp Med 1988; 168:1419-1441.
21. Kurnick JT, Kradin RL, Blumberg R, Schneeberger EE, Boyle LA. Functional characterization of T lymphocytes propagated from human lung carcinomas. Clin Immunol Immunopathol 1986; 38:367-380.
22. Finke JH, Tubbs R, Connelly B, Pontes E, Montie J. Tumor-infiltrating lymphocytes in patients with renal-cell carcinoma. Ann N Y Acad Sci 1988; 532:387-394.
23. Morecki S, Topalian SL, Myers WW, Okrongly D, Okarma TB, Rosenberg SA. Separation and growth of human CD4+ and CD8+ tumor-infiltrating lymphocytes and peripheral blood mononuclear cells by direct positive panning on covalently attached monoclonal antibody-coated flasks. J Biol Resp Mod 1990; 9:463-474.
24. Letessier E, Heo DS, Okarma T, Johnson JT, Herberman RB, Whiteside TL. Enrichment in tumor-reactive CD8+ T lymphocytes by positive selection from the blood and lymph nodes of patients with head and neck cancer. Cancer Res 1991; 51:3891-3899.
25. Itoh K, Shiba KJ, Shimizu Y, Suzuki S, Kamagal K. Generation of activated killer (AK) cells by recombinant interleukin-2 (rIL-2) in collaboration with interferon γ (IFN-γ). J Immunol 1985; 134:3124-3129.
26. Wang YL, Si L, Kanbour A, Herberman

RB, Whiteside TL. Lymphocytes infiltrating human ovarian tumors. Synergy between tumor necrosis factor α and interleukin 2 in the generation of CD8+ effectors from tumor-infiltrating lymphocytes. Cancer Res 1989; 49:5979-5985.
27. Ioannides CG, Platsoucas CD, Rashed S, Wharton JT, Edwards CL, Freedman RS. Tumor cytolysis by lymphocytes infiltrating ovarian malignant ascites. Cancer Res 1991; 51:4257-4265.
28. Owen-Shaub LE, Gutterman JU, Grimm EA. Synergy of tumor necrosis factor and interleukin 2 in the activation of human cytotoxic lymphocytes: Effect of tumor necrosis factorα and interleukin 2 in the generation of human lymphokine-activated killer cell cytotoxicity. Cancer Res 1988; 48:788-792.
29. Lotze MT, Zeh III,H.J., Elder EM, Cai Q, Pippin BA, Rosenstein MM, Whiteside TL, Herberman RB. Use of T-cell growth factors (interleukins 2, 4, 7, 10 and 12) in the evaluation of T-cell reactivity to melanoma. J Immunother 1992; 12:212-217.
30. Giovarelli M, Santoni A, Jemma C, Musso T, Giuffrida AM, Cavello G, Landolfo S, Forni G. Obligatory role of interferon γ induction of lymphokine-activated and T-lymphocyte killer activity, but not in boosting of natural cytotoxicity. J Immunol 1988; 141:2831-2836.
31. Rosenberg SA, Schwarz SL, Spiess P. Combination immunotherapy for cancer: Synergistic antitumor interactions of interleukin 2, α interferon, and tumor-infiltrating lymphocytes. JNCI 1988; 80:1393-1397.
32. Mule JJ, Smith KA, Rosenberg SA. Interleukin-4 (B-cell stimulating factor-1) can mediate the induction of lymphokine-activated killer cell activity directly against fresh tumor cells. J Exp Med 1987; 166:792-804.
33. Rosenberg SA. Lymphokine-activated killer cells: A new approach to immunotherapy of cancer. JNCI 1985; 75:595-603.
34. Kawakami Y, Rosenberg SA, Lotze MT. Interleukin 4 promotes the growth of tumor-infiltrating lymphocytes cytotoxic for human autologous melanoma. J Exp Med 1988; 168:2183-2191.
35. Ranges GE, Figari IS, Espevik T, Palladino MA,Jr. Inhibition of cytotoxic T-cell development by transforming growth factor β and reversal by recombinant tumor necrosis factor α. J Exp Med 1987; 166:991-998.
36. Stotter H, Wiebke EA, Tomita S, Belldegrun A, Topalian S, Rosenberg SA, Lotze MT. Cytokines alter target cell susceptibility to lysis. II. Evaluation of tumor-infiltrating lymphocytes. J Immunol 1989; 141:1767-1773.
37. Jung TT, Berlinger NT, Juhn SK. Prostaglandins in squamous cell carcinoma of the head and neck: A preliminary study. Laryngoscope 1985; 95:307-312.
38. Bodmer S, Strommer K, Frei K, Siepl C, deTribolet N, Heid I, Fontana A. Immunosuppression and transforming growth factor-β in glioblastoma. J Immunol 1989; 143:3222-3229.
39. Snyderman CH, Klapan I, Heo DS, Wagner R, Johnson JT, Whiteside TL. In vitro production of prostaglandin E2 by squamous cell carcinoma of the head and neck. Arch Otolaryngol Head Neck Surg 1993; In press.
40. DeVries JE, Spits H. Cloned human cytotoxic T lymphocyte (CTL) lines reactive with autologous melanoma cells. I. In vitro generation, isolation and analysis of phenotype and specificity. J Immunol 1984; 132:510-519.
41. Knuth A, Danowski B, Oettgen HF, Old LG. T-cell-mediated cytotoxicity against autologous malignant melanoma: Analysis with interleukin-2-dependent T-cell cultures. PNAS USA 1984; 81:3511-3515.
42. Hom SS, Topalian SL, Simonis T, Mancini M, Rosenberg SA. Common expression of melanoma tumor-associated antigens recognized by human tumor-infiltrating lymphocytes: Analysis by human lymphocyte antigen restriction. J Immunother 1991; 10:153-164.
43. Boon T. Tumor antigens recognized by cytolytic T lymphocytes: Present perspectives for specific immunotherapy. Int J Cancer 1993; 54:177-180.
44. Ruiter DJ, Bergman W, Welvaart K, Scheffer E, van Vloten WA, Russo C, Ferrone S. Immunohistochemical analysis of malignant melanomas and nevocellular nevi with monoclonal antibodies to distinct

monomorphic determinants of HLA antigens. Cancer Res 1984; 44:3930-3935.
45. Guerry D, Alexander MA, Herlyn MF, Zehngebot LM, Mitchell KF, Zmijewski CM, Lusk EJ. HLA-DR histocompatibility leukocyte antigens permit cultured human melanoma cells from early but not advanced disease to stimulate autologous lymphocytes. J Clin Invest 1984; 73:267-271.
46. Alexander MA, Bennicelli J, Guerry D. Defective antigen presentation by human melanoma cell lines cultured from advanced, but not biologically early, disease. J Immunol 1989; 142:4070-4078.
47. Yasumura S, Hirabayashi H, Schwartz DR, Toso JF, Johnson JT, Herberman RB, Whiteside TL. Human cytotoxic T-cell lines with restricted specificity for squamous cell carcinoma of the head and neck. Cancer Res 1993; 53:1461-1468.
48. Parmiani G, Anichini A, Fossati G. Cellular immune response against autologous human malignant melanoma: are in vitro studies providing a framework for a more effective immunotherapy? JNCI 1990; 82:361-370.
49. Anichini A, Fossati G, Parmiani G. Clonal analysis of the cytolytic T-cell response to human tumors. Immunol Today 1987; 8:385-389.
50. Alexander J, Rayman P, Edinger M, Connelly R, Tubbs R, Bukowski R, Pontes E, Finke J. TIL from renal-cell carcinoma: Restimulation with tumor influences proliferation and cytolytic activity. Int J Cancer 1990; 45:119-124.
51. Koo AS, Tso C-L, Peyret SC, deKernion JB, Belldegrun A. Autologous tumor-specific cytotoxicity of tumor-infiltrating lymphocytes derived from human renal cell carcinoma. J Immunother 1991; 10:347-354.
52. Skornick Y, Topalian S, Rosenberg SA. Comparative studies of the long-term growth of lymphocytes from tumor infiltrates, tumor-draining lymph nodes, and peripheral blood by repeated in vitro stimulation with autologous tumor. J Biol Resp Mod 1990; 9:431-438.
53. van der Bruggen P, Traversari C, Chomez P, Lurquin C, de Plaen E, Van den Eynde B, Knuth A, Boon T. A gene encoding an antigen recognized by cytolytic T lymphocytes on a human melanoma. Science 1991; 254:1643-1647.
54. Finke JH, Rayman P, Edinger M, Tubbs RR, Stanley J, Klein E, Bukowski R. Characterization of a human renal cell carcinoma specific cytotoxic CD8+ T-cell line. J Immunol 1991; 11:1-11.
55. Shimizu Y, Weidmann E, Iwatsuki S, Herberman RB, Whiteside TL. Characterization of human autotumor-reactive T-cell clones obtained from tumor-infiltrating lymphocytes in liver metastasis of gastric carcinoma. Cancer Res 1991; 51:6153-6162.
56. Wolfel T, Klehmann E, Muller C, Schutt KH, Meyer zum Buschenfelde KH, Knuth A. Lysis of human melanoma cells by autologous cytolytic T-cell clones: Identification of human histocompatibility leukocyte antigen A2 as a restriction element for three different antigens. J Exp Med 1989; 170:797-810.
57. Crowley NJ, Darrow TL, Quinn-Aleen MA, Seigler HF. MHC-restricted recognition of autologous melanoma by tumor-specific cytotoxic T cells: Evidence for restriction by a dominant HLA-A allele. J Immunol 1991; 146:1692-1699.
58. Traversari C, van der Bruggen P, Luescher IF, Lurquin C, Chomez P, Van Pel A, de Plaen E, Amar-Costesec A, Boon T. A nonapeptide encoded by human gene MAGE-1 is recognized on HLA-A1 by cytolytic T lymphocytes directed against tumor antigen MZ2-E. J Exp Med 1992; 176:1453-1457.
59. Weber JS, Rosenberg SA. Effects of murine tumor class I major histocompatibility complex expression on antitumor activity of tumor-infiltrating lymphocytes. JNCI 1990; 82:755-761.
60. Bjorkman PJ, Saper MA, Samraoui B, Bennett WS, Strominger JL, Wiley DC. The foreign antigen binding site and T-cell recognition regions of class I histocompatibility antigens. Nature 1987; 332:512-518.
61. Townsend A, Rothband J, Gotch F, Bahadur G, Wraith D, McMichael A. The epitopes of influenza nucleoprotein recognized by cytotoxic T lymphocytes can be defined with short synthetic peptides. Cell 1986; 44:959-968.

62. Kawakami Y, Zakut R, Topalian SL, Stotter H, Rosenberg SA. Shared human melanoma antigens. Recognition by tumor-infiltrating lymphocytes in HLA-A2.1-transfected melanomas. J Immunol 1992; 148:638-643.
63. Traversari C, van der Bruggen P, Van den Eynde B, Hainaut P, Lemoine C, Ohta N, Boon T. Transfection and expression of a gene coding for human melanoma antigen recognized by autologous cytolytic T lymphocytes. Immunogenetics 1992; 35:145-152.
64. Barnd DL, Lamm S, Metzgar RS, Finn OJ. Specific, major histocompatibility complex-unrestricted recognition of tumor-ass mucins by human cytotoxic T cells. PNAS USA 1989; 86:7159-7163.
65. Barnd D, Kerr L, Metzgar RS, Finn OJ. Tumor specific cytotoxic T-cell lines generated from tumor-draining lymph node infiltrate. Transpl Proc 1988; 20:339-341.
66. Jerome KR, Barnd DL, Bendt KM, Bower CM, Taylor-Papadimitriou J, McKendzie IF, Bast Jr, RC, Finn OJ. Cytotoxic T-lymphocytes derived from patients with breast adenocarcinoma recognize an epitope present on the protein core of a mucin molecule preferentially expressed by malignant cells. Cancer Res 1991; 51:2908-2916.
67. Ioannides CG, Fisk B, Jerome KR, Irimura T, Freedman RS, Finn OJ. Cytotoxic T cells isolated from ovarian tumor-infiltrating lymphocytes can recognize tumor mucins. Proc AACR 1991; 33:A1884.
68. Shimizu Y, Iwatsuki S, Herberman RB, Whiteside TL. Clonal analysis of tumor-infiltrating lymphocytes from human primary and metastatic liver tumors. Int J Cancer 1990; 46:878-883.
69. Miescher S, Whiteside TL, Moretta L, Von Fliedner V. Clonal and frequency analyses of tumor-infiltrating T lymphocytes from human solid tumors. J Immunol 1987; 138:4004-4011.
70. Moretta A, Pantaleo G, Moretta L, Cerottini JC, Mingari MC. Direct demonstration of the clonogenic potential of every human peripheral blood T cells. Clonal analysis of HLA-DR expression and cytolytic activity. J Exp Med 1983; 157:743-754.
71. Anichini A, Fossati G, Parmiani G. Heterogeneity of clones from a human metastatic melanoma detected by autologous cytotoxic T lymphocyte clones. J Exp Med 1986; 163:215-220.
72. Fossati G, Anichini A, Squarcina P, Mazzocchi A, Parmiani G. Proliferative and/or cytotoxic activity of lymphocyte clones to autologous human melanoma. Int J Cancer 1988; 42:239-245.
73. Mukherji B, Guha A, Chakraborty NG, Sivanandham M, Nashed AL, Sporn JR, Ergin MT. Clonal analysis of cytotoxic and regulatory T-cell responses against human melanoma. J Exp Med 1989; 169:1961-1976.
74. Yasumura S, Weidmann E, Hirabayashi H, Johnson JT, Herberman RB, Whiteside TL. HLA-A2 and T-cell receptor restriction of cytotoxic T lymphocytes reactive with human squamous cell carcinoma of the head and neck. Arch Otolaryngol Head Neck Surg 1993; In press.
75. Darrow TL, Slingluff Jr,C.L., Siegler HF. The role of HLA class I antigens in recognition of melanoma cells by tumor-specific cytotoxic T lymphocytes. J Immunol 1989; 142:3329-3335.
76. Belldegrun A, Kasid A, Uppenkamp M, Rosenberg SA. Lymphokine mRNA profile and functional analysis of a human CD4+ clone with unique antitumor specificity isolated from renal cell carcinoma ascitic fluid. Cancer Immunol Immunother 1990; 31:1-10.
77. Schwartzentruber DJ, Topalian SL, Mancini M, Rosenberg SA. Specific release of granulocyte-macrophage colony-stimulating factor, tumor necrosis factor-α, and IFN-γ by human tumor-infiltrating lymphocytes after autologous tumor stimulation. J Immunol 1991; 146:3674-3681.
78. Romagniani S. Human TH1 and TH2: Doubt no more. Immunol Today 1991; 12:256-257.
79. Paliard X, deWaal MR, Yssel H, Blanchard D, Chretien I, Abrams J, deVries J, Spits H. Simultaneous production of IL-2, IL-4 and IFN-γ by activated human CD4+ and CD8+ T-cell clones. J Immunol 1988; 141:849-855.
80. Hom SS, Schwartzentruber DJ, Rosenberg SA, Topalian SL. Specific release of cytokines by lymphocytes infiltrating human melanomas in response to shared melanoma

antigens. J Immunother 1993; 13:18-30.
81. Barth Jr,R.J., Mule JJ, Asher AL, Sanda MG, Rosenberg SA. Identification of unique murine tumor associated antigens by tumor-infiltrating lymphocytes using tumor specific secretion of interferon-γ and tumor necrosis factor. J Immunol Methods 1991; 140:269-279.
82. Barth RJ, Mule JJ, Spiess PJ, Rosenberg SA. Interferon γ and tumor necrosis factor have a role in tumor regressions mediated by murine CD8+ tumor-infiltrating lymphocytes. J Exp Med 1991; 173:647-658.
83. Ortaldo JR, Mason A, Overton R. Lymphokine-activated killer cells: Analysis of progenitors and effectors. J Exp Med 1986; 164:1193-1205.
84. Cianciolo GJ, Lostrom ME, Tam M, Snyderman R. Murine malignant cells synthesize a 19,000-dalton protein that is physicochemically and antigenically related to the immunosuppressive retroviral protein, P15E. J Exp Med 1983; 158:885-900.
85. Snyderman R, Cianciolo GJ. Immunosuppressive activity of the retroviral envelope protein p15E and its possible relationship to neoplasia. Immunol Today 1984; 5:240-242.
86. Packard BS. Mitogenic stimulation of human tumor-infiltrating lymphocytes by secreted factor(s) from human tumor cell lines. PNAS USA 1990; 87:4058-4062.
87. Rabinowich H, Vitolo D, Altarac S, Herberman RB, Whiteside TL. Role of cytokines in the adoptive immunotherapy of an experimental model of human head and neck cancer by human IL-2-activated natural killer cells. J Immunol 1992; 149:340-349.
88. Uchida A, Moore M. Lysis of fresh human tumor cells by autologous large granular lymphocytes and T-lymphocytes: Two distinct killing activities induced by coculture with autologous tumor. JNCI 1984; 73:1285-1292.
89. Brooks CG, Urdal DL, Henney CS. Lymphokine-driven "differentiation" of cytotoxic T-cell clones into cells with NK-like specificity: correlations with display of membrane macromolecules. Immunol Rev 1983; 72:43-72.
90. Anichini A, Mazzocchi A, Fossati G, Parmiani G. Cytotoxic T lymphocyte clones from peripheral blood and from tumor site detect intratumor heterogeneity of melanoma cells. Analysis of specificity and mechanisms of interaction. J Immunol 1989; 142:3692-3701.
91. Moy PM, Holmes EC, Golub SH. Depression of natural killer cytotoxic activity in lymphocytes infiltrating human pulmonary tumors. Cancer Res 1985; 45:57-60.
92. Eremin O, Coombs RRA, Ashby J. Lymphocytes infiltrating human breast cancers lack K-cell activity and show low levels of NK-cell activity. Br J Cancer 1981; 44:166-175.
93. Introna M, Allavena P, Biondi A, Colombo N, Villa A, Mantovani A. Defective natural killer activity within human ovarian tumors: Low numbers of morphologically defined effectors present in situ. JNCI 1983; 70:21-26.
94. Weidmann E, Elder EM, Trucco M, Lotze MT, Whiteside TL. Usage of T-cell receptor V β chain genes in fresh and cultured tumor-infiltrating lymphocytes from human melanoma. Int J Cancer 1993; 54:383-390.
95. Nitta T, Oksenberg JR, Rao NA, Steinman L. Predominant expression of T-cell receptor V α 7 in tumor-infiltrating lymphocytes of uveal melanoma. Science 1990; 249:672-674.
96. Van den Eynde B, Hainaut P, Herin M, Knuth A, Lemoine C, Weynants P, van der Bruggen P, Fauchet R, Boon T. Presence on a human melanoma of multiple antigens recognized by autologous CTL. Int J Cancer 1989; 44:634-640.
97. Notter M, Schirrmacher V. Tumor-specific T-cell clones recognize different protein determinants of autologous human malignant melanoma cells. Int J Cancer 1990; 45:834-841.
98. Barth RJ, Jr., Bock SN, Mule JJ, Rosenberg SA. Unique murine tumor-associated antigens identified by tumor-infiltrating lymphocytes. J Immunol 1990; 144:1531-1537.
99. Shu S, Chou T, Sakai K. Lymphocytes generated by in vivo priming and in vitro sensitization demonstrate therapeutic efficacy against a murine tumor that lacks apparent immunogenicity. J Immunol 1989; 143:740-748.

CHAPTER 7

TIL and Their Role in Tumor Surveillance and Progression

One of the fundamental questions about involvement of the immune system in surveillance against the emerging tumors and control of tumor progression and metastasis concerns the mechanism of recognition of human AuTu by T cells. The concept of T-cell mediated tumor surveillance implies that mature T cells in the periphery are able to detect antigenic changes that occur on the surface of tissue cells, which have entered the process of transition from a normal to premalignant to malignant state. Such recognition should ultimately lead to both elimination of tumor cells and generation of immunologic memory mediated by T cells. This concept also implies that AuTu-reactive T cells are present in patients with cancer and that TAA are immunogenic, i.e., are able to evoke memory T-cell responses. In addition to memory, generation of protective immunity against tumor is expected to be a part of effective antitumor responses.

TUMOR-SPECIFIC T CELLS IN SURVEILLANCE

The role of T cells in surveillance against human solid tumors has been questioned for several good reasons in recent years. First, T-cell mediated responses to putative human TAA have been difficult to demonstrate. Although T cells or T-cell clones with specificity for TAA have been occasionally isolated from the peripheral blood or TIL of patients with melanoma or RCC and established in culture,[1-3] existence of such T-cell clones in most of the other human solid tumors remains uncertain. Second, evidence for the ability of primary or metastatic human tumors to evoke T-cell responses is limited, mostly because antigenic changes that occur on the tumor cell surface seem to be quantitative rather than qualitative and because antigenic modulation often appears to interfere with the Ag presentation on the surface of tumor cells.[4] Third, the requirements for Ag presentation to T cells are rigidly defined, and it is likely that many human tumors or TAA fail to meet these requirements for various reasons. This suggests that although TAA may be immunogenic, and, thus, are recognized by the appropriate immune cells, the process of Ag presentation and recognition is defective in tumor-bearing hosts so that protective immunity against the tumor cannot be generated. Evidence has accumulated recently in support of this possibility, at least in murine tumor-bearing hosts.[5,6] In fact, in only a few experimental tumor model systems, involving chemically-induced or viral tumors, has evidence for protective immunity been obtained.[7] Last, but not least, tumors have evolved ways to escape immune recognition, and as discussed in Chapter 5, the ability to release immunosuppressive factors directed at T cells may be one mechanism of such escape. Perhaps the key issues in respect to tumor surveillance are those of timing and localization of T-cell responses. By the time a TAA is presented as required and a local T-cell response ensues, the tumor may have metastasized to another site or undergone further antigenic modification. Thus, T cells, which are a relatively late component of the immune response, may not be as effective a surveillance mechanism against tumor growth or metastasis as is generally assumed, and other non-MHC-restricted immune cells, e.g., NK cells, may be primarily involved in the process of surveillance. Nevertheless, it is well known that lymphomas[8] and certain solid tumors[9] are more frequent in immunosuppressed or immunodeficient individuals than in immunologically normal populations, and the role of AuTu-specific T cells or other subsets of immune cells in control of cancer development remains to be elucidated.

TUMOR-SPECIFIC T CELLS AND CONTROL OF TUMOR GROWTH

While the role of AuTu-specific T cells in surveillance against human solid tumors remains uncertain, there is some evidence that such T cells are present in tumor-bearing hosts and that they may be involved in the regulation of tumor growth. Infiltrations of activated T cells into the tumor seem to indicate that a patient's immune system is able to develop a local antitumor response. Whether this response is mediated by inflammatory, non-MHC-restricted T cells or by MHC-restricted AuTu-specific T cells remains to be determined. Most likely, both nonspecific and AuTu-specific T cells contribute to the local antitumor response. However, these TIL appear to be largely ineffective in limiting tumor progression.

Surprisingly, when fresh TIL-T isolated from human solid tumors were tested for antitumor function in in vitro assays, they showed poor cytotoxicity against AuTu or other tumor targets and failed to proliferate in response to T-cell mitogens and other stimuli (see Chapter 5). This state of functional unresponsiveness could, however, be reversed, because the same cells after culture in the presence of cytokines and irradiated AuTu became able to proliferate and mediate cytotoxicity.[1,10-12] Moreover, cultured TIL adoptively transferred to cancer patients with metastatic disease have been reported to induce partial or complete clinical responses in a proportion of these patients.[13] To explain this apparent paradox of phenotypically-activated yet functionally-paralyzed tumor-derived T cells, recent studies have focused on a better understanding of T cell interactions with AuTu. A complex picture of events has emerged, which indicates that the immune response at the tumor site involves specific Ag recognition by T cells, activation, lymphokine secretion, amplification of the response, and the subsequent inflammatory phase, and that tumor actively participates in modulating this response by secretion of a variety of factors with powerful effects on the immune and other cells.[14-17]

RECOGNITION OF TAA BY T CELLS

It has been established that T cells recognize Ags as short peptides bound to the MHC molecules only when these peptides are presented on the surface of target cells or APC. Due to a high degree of polymorphism in the MHC, individual T cells recognize the peptide Ags in association with a particular MHC allelic product, a phenomenon referred to as the MHC restriction.[18] With the notable exception of mucin-reactive T cells,[19] most T cells apparently follow this rule. Polymorphic epithelial mucins (PEM) contain a polypeptide core, which is unglycosylated or poorly glycosylated in tumor cells.[20] The repeating nonapeptide units of the core peptide can directly bind to the TcR and activate $CD8^+$ T cells. This property resembles the ability of T-cell-independent Ags to activate B cells.

The current view of tumor Ag recognition is that tumor-derived peptides, which have a minimum of nine amino acids in length, are recognized by $CD8^+$ cells[21,22] and somewhat longer peptides (16-18 residues) are recognized by CD4⁺ cells.[23,24] Many TAA expressed on human tumors are a result of point mutations affecting "household" genes expressed in all normal cells. These mutations often generate strong new Ags recognized by CTL.[25-27] Some of these mutations confer upon a peptide or epitope the ability to bind a class I MHC molecule and, thus, the ability to be recognized by CTL.[27,28] Others confer a new epitope or a different motif to the antigenic peptide, leading to its recognition by a new set of CTL.[27] In other cases, activation of a silent gene occurs as a result of transformation. The best characterized of human TAA able to induce CTL response is a melanoma Ag (MZ2-E) coded by MAGE-1 gene and presented by HLA-A1.[29,30] This Ag is expressed on tumor cells of about 40% of patients with melanoma.[27] The MAGE-1-encoded antigenic peptide that binds to HLA-A1 has been identified as a nonapeptide. Whatever is the nature of TAA recognized by CTL, the key characteristics of T-cell responses to TAA are specificity and memory. This means that whenever the Ag-reactive T-cell clone recognizes a unique epitope via the TcR, it responds by proliferation, lymphokine secretion, and in the case of CTL, by lysis of the targets expressing this epitope and generation of long-lived memory T cells.

Expression of Ags on tumor cells or on APC provides a ligand for the TcR on tumor-reactive T cells. However, following the initial event of Ag recognition, additional signals are required to trigger the T cell.[31] Thus, recognition by the AuTu-specific T cell of an Ag expressed in the context of the class I MHC Ags is followed by transduction of signals delivered via the TcR that result in induction or up-regulation of lymphokine receptors and in cytokine production. Various surface molecules on tumor or accessory cells are known to enhance Ag recognition (e.g., CD8, CD4, LFA-1, class I or class II MHC Ags or ICAM-1). Inducible signals necessary for development of effector T-cell function might involve the release of soluble cytokines and interactions of CD28 on T-cells with B7 Ag on B cells or macrophages.[31-33] Since tumor recognition is Ag-specific and class I MHC-restricted, lymphokine secretion is currently considered to be an indicator of specific recognition.[34,35] Recent evidence has suggested that the TcR has the capacity of differential signalling, i.e., that cytokine production can be dissociated from other T-cell functions.[36] It remains unclear whether induction or up-regulation of CTL cytotoxicity reflects solely the dependence on the TcR-mediated activation of cytokine genes because the outcome of the interaction between the T cell and Ag requires the participation of APC.[31] This raises the question whether the AuTu can provide adequate accessory signals for activation of the CTL which, in fact, are expected to recognize the Ag on its surface. Therefore, if Ag presentation by the tumor fails to provide the accessory signals needed by T cells, either an incomplete activation process or a generalized state of unresponsiveness may result. This is in agreement with the hypothesis formulated by Bretscher and Cohn that defective Ag recognition may lead to long-lasting inactivation of T cells.[37,38] On the other hand, nonlymphoid cells, e.g., tumor-infiltrating macrophages, could function as APC in the tumor microenvironment. It has also been demonstrated, however, that these macrophages may be functionally defective[39,40] and thus perhaps unable to adequately present Ags. High concentrations of tumor Ags in the tumor microenvironment in the absence of functional APC may lead to Ag-specific inactivation of TIL analogous with findings in other experimental systems.[41,42] The fact that, in many instances, lymphocytes infiltrating human tumors are outnumbered by tumor cells provides additional support for this hypothesis. It has been demonstrated that T cells stimulated with low concentrations of Ag may fail to proliferate.[38] Studies by Schwartz and colleagues tentatively defined the state of anergy (unresponsiveness) of mature T cells as the inability of Ag-stimulated T cells to up-regulate IL-2R, to release IL-2 and to proliferate in response to the specific Ag. The state of anergy can be reversed by using high concentrations of IL-2 in culture.[38] It is of interest to note that freshly isolated TIL or LNL from tumor-involved lymph nodes are often unresponsive in vitro to various antigenic stimuli, including AuTu, and that this unresponsiveness may be reversed in the presence of IL-2 and APC.[43]

TAA AS SELF-ANTIGENS

The nature of Ags or epitopes recognized by T cells on tumor remains mostly undefined. In some cases, these Ags are mutated self-products[7,27] or perhaps overexpressed oncogenes.[28,44] In general, T cells are capable of distinguishing mutated peptides with exquisite specificity, e.g., at the level of one nonconservative amino acid substitution.[27] However, T cells fail to respond to unaltered self-products, the phenomenon referred to as self-tolerance.[45] Autoreactive T-cell clones are silenced or eliminated before acquiring immunologic competence, generally early in the process of maturation in the thymus.[46,47] If TAA are viewed as expression of self, then it could be expected that no specific T- or B-cell responses can be mounted against malignant cells. Such is not the case, however, because both antibodies and AuTu reactive T cells have been identified in patients with tumors. It must, therefore, be accepted that either DNA mutations or activation of normally silent genes which accompany malignant transformation result in expression on the surface of tumor cells of novel, mutated or overexpressed, cellular proteins. Immune cells are expected to recognize such altered cellular products, unless these products resemble normal self-proteins. In such a case, it is possible that tumor-reactive T cells may be eliminated or deleted because they express TcR for self-proteins.

It has recently been demonstrated that clonal deletion appears not to be restricted to immature T cells but can be the end-point of certain immune responses, e.g., to superantigens.[47] Selective elimination of V β 2^+ cells has been recently reported in mice bearing preneoplastic lesions.[48] The fact that certain of the tumor-associated proteins are normally expressed only during fetal development (i.e., are oncofetal Ags) further supports the hypothesis that self-reactive immune cell clones recognizing these Ags are eliminated during development. Thus, the lack of immune responses to tumor cells might be a result of clonal deletion which could be viewed as an attempt to eliminate self-reactive T cells. Similarly, immunosuppression present in the tumor microenvironment could serve the same purpose, with subsequent elimination of auto-immune responses but also of tumor-reactive T-cell clones.

UP-REGULATION OF ANTITUMOR RESPONSES

Various approaches have been tried to overcome unresponsiveness of antitumor effector cells and to increase specific as well as nonspecific antitumor responses in patients with cancer.[49,50] The former goal can be achieved by immunization with native or synthetic tumor-associated peptides,[27] while the latter approach largely depends on the clinical use of cytokines.[51] Among many recombinant cytokines that are available, IL-2 has been utilized most extensively and, today, it is the only cytokine approved for therapy of melanoma and RCC. The effects of systemic or locoregional delivery of IL-2 on the number or function of TIL in patients with cancer have been evaluated in a handful of studies.[52-55] Using immunohistology, Rubin and colleagues have compared tumor tissues obtained pre- and posttherapy from 48 patients with advanced malignancies treated with systemic IL-2 alone or in combination with cyclophosphamide and/or adoptively-transferred effector cells.[53] Their findings indicated that clinical responses to IL-2-based immunotherapy were associated with T-cell as well as macrophage infiltrations of the tumor site. Similarly, we have demonstrated significant accumulation of activated T and NK cells at the tumor site and up-regulation of their antitumor activity as a result of perilesional IL-2 administration to patients with inoperable SCCHN.[55] These examples suggest that therapy with IL-2 induces both local and systemic changes in the number and function of antitumor effector cells. In addition, recent discovery of IL-2R able to bind IL-2 on human carcinomas[56,57] and melanomas,[58] and the observation that IL-2 might directly inhibit tumor growth upon binding to these IL-2R suggests that IL-2 is not only immunostimulatory, but that it has cytostatic effects on at least some tumors.

It has been suggested that both acute and chronic inflammatory cells play a crucial role in local antitumor responses.[59] Activation of these inflammatory cells by locally available cytokines leads to granulocyte-T-lymphocyte cross-talk, which appears to be essential for tumor rejection.[59] Delivery of exogenous cytokines or induction of cytokine production in the tumor environment appears to alter the natural tumor-host interactions and may shift the immune balance in favor of the host.[60] In fact, this rationale has been the basis for gene therapy of cancer with tumor cells transfected with cytokine genes.[61-63] Cytokine therapy, particularly locoregional therapy, may be effective in altering the tumor microenvironment and in changing intrinsic properties of tumor cells, thereby making them more susceptible to immune effector cells present at the tumor site.[55]

SUMMARY

Evidence has accumulated for the presence of specific AuTu effector T cells among TIL in patients with cancer. However, it remains unclear why AuTu-specific T cells able to recognize TAA or peptides are ineffective in control of tumor progression. Interactions between TIL and tumor cells are complex, and it is surmised that immunosuppression, which is commonly seen in the tumor microenvironment is responsible, at least in part, for down-regulation of the AuTu-specific T-cell response. This down-regulation may represent an attempt by the host to dampen or control self-reactivity rather than facilitate escape of the tumor from immune surveillance. In fact, aside from well-documented predisposition for development of cancer in immunosuppressed or immunodeficient individuals, no convincing evidence for the role of AuTu-reactive T cells in surveillance against malignancy exists today. AuTu-specific or nonspecific T cells accumulating at the site of tumor growth may be involved, however, in regulation of tumor growth. This TIL-mediated regulation involves mutual T-cell-tumor cell interactions, and it may sometimes benefit the tumor rather than the host. A better understanding of T-cell-tumor interactions is necessary to overcome tumor-induced suppression of immune cells. To an extent, up-regulation of local antitumor immune responses can be achieved through therapeutic delivery of cytokines to the tumor site. It is likely that future efforts will be directed at reducing or eliminating tumor-mediated immunosuppression of T-cell responses.

REFERENCES

1. Topalian SL, Solomon D, Rosenberg SA. Tumor-specific cytolysis by lymphocytes infiltrating human melanomas. J Immunol 1989; 142:3714-3724.
2. Mukherji B, Guha A, Chakraborty NG, Sivanandham M, Nashed AL, Sporn JR, Ergin MT. Clonal analysis of cytotoxic and regulatory T-cell responses against human melanoma. J Exp Med 1989; 169:1961-1976.
3. Finke JH, Rayman P, Edinger M, Tubbs RR, Stanley J, Klein E, Bukowski R. Characterization of a human renal cell carcinoma specific cytotoxic CD8+ T-cell line. J Immunol 1991; 11:1-11.
4. Old LJ. Cancer Immunology. The search for specificity. Cancer Res 1981; 41:361-375.
5. Loeffler CM, Smyth MJ, Longo DL, Kopp WC, Harvey LK, Tribble HR, Tase JE, Urba WJ, Leonard AS, Young HA, Ochoa AC. Immunoregulation in cancer-bearing hosts. Down-regulation of gene expression and cytotoxic function in CD8+ T cells. J Immunol 1992; 149:949-956.
6. Mizoguchi H, O'Shea JJ, Longo DL, Loeffler CM, McVicar DW, Ochoa AC. Alterations in signal transduction molecules in T lymphocytes from tumor-bearing mice. Science 1992; 258:1795-1798.
7. Urban JL, Schriber H. Tumor antigens. Ann Rev Immunol 1992; 10:617-644.
8. Ho M, Jaffe R, Miller G, Breinig MK, Dummer JS, Makowka L, Atchison RW, Karrer F, Nalesnik MA, Starzl TE. The frequency of Epstein-Barr virus infection and associated lymphoproliferative syndrome after transplantation and its manifestation in

children. Transplantation 1988; 45:719-727.
9. Penn I. Cancers complicating organ transplantation. NEJM 1990; 323:1767-1769.
10. Whiteside TL, Heo DS, Takagi S, Johnson JT, Iwatsuki S, Herberman RB. Cytotoxic antitumor effector cells in long-term cultures of human tumor-infiltrating lymphocytes in recombinant IL-2. Cancer Immunol Immunother 1988; 26:1-10.
11. Ioannides CG, Platsoucas CD, Rashed S, Wharton JT, Edwards CL, Freedman RS. Tumor cytolysis by lymphocytes infiltrating ovarian malignant ascites. Cancer Res 1991; 51:4257-4265.
12. Itoh K, Platsoucas CD, Balch CM. Autologous tumor-specific cytotoxic T lymphocytes in the infiltrate of human metastatic melanomas. Activation by interleukin 2 and autologous tumor cells, and involvement of the T-cell receptor. J Exp Med 1988; 168:1419-1441.
13. Rosenberg SA, Packard BS, Aebersold PM, Solomon D, Topalian SL, Toy ST, Simon P, Lotze MT, Yang JC, Seipp CA, Simpson C, Carter C, Bock S, Schwartzentruber D, Wei JP, White DE. Use of tumor-infiltrating lymphocytes and interleukin-2 in the immunotherapy of patients with metastatic melanoma. A preliminary report. N Engl J Med 1988; 319:1676-1680.
14. Snyderman R, Cianciolo GJ. Immunosuppressive activity of the retroviral envelope protein p15E and its possible relationship to neoplasia. Immunol Today 1984; 5:240-242.
15. Putnam JB, Roth JA. Identification and characterization of a tumor-derived immunosuppressive glycoprotein from murine melanoma K-1735. Cancer Immunol Immunother 1985; 19:90-100.
16. Rabinowich H, Vitolo D, Altarac S, Herberman RB, Whiteside TL. Role of cytokines in the adoptive immunotherapy of an experimental model of human head and neck cancer by human IL-2-activated natural killer cells. J Immunol 1992; 149:340-349.
17. Packard BS. Mitogenic stimulation of human tumor-infiltrating lymphocytes by secreted factor(s) from human tumor cell lines. PNAS USA 1990; 87:4058-4062.
18. Robbins PA, Lettice LA, Rota P, Santos AJ, Rothbard J, McMichael AJ, Strominger JL. Comparison between two peptide epitopes presented to cytotoxic T lymphocytes by HLA-A2: Evidence for discrete locations within HLA-A2. J Immunol 1988; 143:4098-4103.
19. Barnd DL, Lamm S, Metzgar RS, Finn OJ. Specific, major histocompatibility complex-unrestricted recognition of tumor-ass mucins by human cytotoxic T cells. PNAS USA 1989; 86:7159-7163.
20. Jerome KR, Barnd DL, Bendt KM, Bower CM, Taylor-Papadimitriou J, McKendzie IF, Bast RC Jr, Finn OJ. Cytotoxic T-lymphocytes derived from patients with breast adenocarcinoma recognize an epitope present on the protein core of a mucin molecule preferentially expressed by malignant cells. Cancer Res 1991; 51:2908-2916.
21. Van-Bleek GM, Nathenson SG. Isolation of an endogenously processed immunodominant viral peptide from the class I H-2Kb molecule. Nature 1990; 348:213-216.
22. Falk K, Rotzschke O, Deres K, Metzger J, Jung G, Rammensee HG. Identification of naturally processed viral nonapeptides allows their quantification in infected cells and suggests an allele-specific T-cell epitope forecast. J Exp Med 1991; 174:425-434.
23. Rudensky AY, Preston-Hurlburt P, Hong SC, Barlow A, Janeway J Jr. Sequence analysis of peptides bound to MHC class II molecules. Nature 1991; 353:622-627.
24. Sadegh-Nasseri S, Germain RN. A role for peptide in determining MHC class II structure. Nature 1991; 353:167-170.
25. DePlaen E, Lurquin C, Van Pel A, Mariame B, Szikora J, Wolfel T, Sibille C, Chomez P, Boon T. Tum-variants of mouse mastocytoma P815. IX. Cloning of the gene of tum-antigen P91A and identification of the tum-mutation. PNAS USA 1988; 85:2274-2278.
26. Sibille C, Chomez P, Wildmann C, Van Pel A, de Plaen E, Maryanski J, De Bergeyck V, Boon T. Structure of the gene of tum-transplantation antigen P198: A point mutation generates a new antigenic peptide. J Exp Med 1990; 172:35-45.
27. Boon T. Tumor antigens recognized by cytolytic T lymphocytes: Present perspectives for specific immunotherapy. Int J

Cancer 1993; 54:177-180.
28. Jung S, Schluesner HJ. Human T lymphocytes recognize a peptide of single point-mutated, oncogenic ras proteins. J Exp Med 1991; 173:273-276.
29. van der Bruggen P, Traversari C, Chomez P, Lurquin C, de Plaen E, Van den Eynde B, Knuth A, Boon T. A gene encoding an antigen recognized by cytolytic T lymphocytes on a human melanoma. Science 1991; 254:1643-1647.
30. Traversari C, van der Bruggen P, Luescher IF, Lurquin C, Chomez P, Van Pel A, de Plaen E, Amar-Costesec A, Boon T. A nonapeptide encoded by human gene MAGE-1 is recognized on HLA-A1 by cytolytic T lymphocytes directed against tumor antigen MZ2-E. J Exp Med 1992; 176:1453-1457.
31. Weaver CT, Unanue ER. The co-stimulatory function of antigen-presenting cells. Immunol Today 1990; 11:49-55.
32. Harding FA, McArthur JG, Gross JA, Raulet DH, Allison JP. CD28-mediated signalling co-stimulates murine T cells and prevents induction of anergy in T-cell clones. Nature 1992; 356:607-609.
33. Townsend SE, Allison JP. Tumor rejection after direct co-stimulation of CD8+ T cells by B7-transfected melanoma cells. Science 1993; 259:368-370.
34. Schwartzentruber DJ, Topalian SL, Mancini M, Rosenberg SA. Specific release of granulocyte-macrophage colony-stimulating factor, tumor necrosis factor-α, and IFN-γ by human tumor-infiltrating lymphocytes after autologous tumor stimulation. J Immunol 1991; 146:3674-3681.
35. Hom SS, Schwartzentruber DJ, Rosenberg SA, Topalian SL. Specific release of cytokines by lymphocytes infiltrating human melanomas in response to shared melanoma antigens. J Immunother 1993; 13:18-30.
36. Otten GR, Germain RN. Split anergy in a CD8+ T cell: Receptor-dependent cytolysis in the absence of interleukin-2 production. Science 1991; 251:1228-1231.
37. Bretscher P, Cohn M. A theory of self-nonself discrimination. Science 1970; 169:1042-1049.
38. Schwartz RH. A cell culture model for T lymphocyte clonal anergy. Science 1990; 248:1349-1356.
39. Erroi A, Casali B, Donati MB, Mantovani A, Semeraro N. Mouse tumor-associated macrophages do not generate procoagulant activity in response to different stimuli. Int J Cancer 1988; 41:65-68.
40. Mantovani A, Bottazzi B, Colotta F, Sozzani S, Ruco L. The origin and function of tumor-associated macrophages. Immunol Today 1992; 13:265-270.
41. Lamb JR, Feldmann M. Essential requirement for major histocompatibility complex recognition in T-cell tolerance induction. Nature 1984; 308:72-74.
42. Pawelec G, Brocker T, Busch FW, Buhring HJ, Fernandez N, Schneider EM, Wernet P. "Tolerization" of human T-helper cell clones by chronic exposure to alloantigen: Culture conditions dictate autocrine proliferative status but not acquisition of cytotoxic potential and suppressor-induction capacity. J Mol Cell Immunol 1988; 4:21-34.
43. Cozzolino F, Torcia M, Carossino AM, Giordani R, Selli C, Talini G, Reali E, Novelli A, Pistoia V, Ferrarini M. Characterization of cells from invaded lymph nodes in patients with solid tumors. J Exp Med 1987; 166:303-318.
44. Peace DJ, Chen W, Nelson H, Cheever MA. T-cell recognition of transforming proteins encoded by mutated ras proto-oncogenes. J Immunol 1991; 146:2059-2065.
45. Miller JF, Morahan G. Peripheral T-cell tolerance. Ann Rev Immunol 1957; 10:51-69.
46. Kisielow P, Bluthmann H, Staerz UD, Steinmetz M, Von Boehmer H. Tolerance in T-cell receptor transgenic mice involves deletion of non-mature CD4+CD8+ thymocytes. Nature 1988; 333:742-746.
47. Webb S, Morris C, Sprent J. Extrathymic tolerance of mature T cells: Clonal elimination as a consequence of immunity. Cell 1990; 63:1249-1256.
48. Wei WZ, Ficsor-Jacobs R, Tsai SJ, Pauley R. Elimination of V β 2-bearing T cells in BALB/c mice implanted with syngeneic preneoplastic and neoplastic mammary lesions. Cancer Res 1991; 51:3331-3333.
49. Whiteside TL, Herberman RB. Characteristics of natural killer cells and lymphokine-

activated killer cells. Their role in the biology and treatment of human cancer. In: Oettgen HF., ed. Human Cancer Immunology I: Immunology and Allergy Clinics of North America. Philadelphia: W.B. Saunders Co., 1990: 663-704.
50. Mitchell MS. Attempts to optimize active specific immunotherapy for melanoma. Int Rev Immunol 1991; 7:331-347.
51. Borden EC, Sondell PM. Lymphokines and cytokines in cancer treatment immunotherapy realized. Cancer 1990; 65:800-814.
52. Rivoltini L, Gambacorti-Passerini C, Squadrelli-Saraceno M, Grosso MI, Cantu G, Molinari R, Orazi A, Parmiani G. In vivo interleukin 2-induced activation of lymphocyte-activated killer cells and tumor cytotoxic-T cells in cervical lymph nodes of patients with head and neck tumors. Cancer Res 1990; 50:5551-5557.
53. Rubin JT, Elwood LJ, Rosenberg SA, Lotze MT. Immunohistochemical correlates of response to recombinant interleukin 2-based immunotherapy in humans. Cancer Res 1989; 49:7086-7092.
54. Valente G, De Stefani A, Jemma C, Giovarelli M, Geuna M, Cortesina G, Forni G, Palestro G. Infiltrating leukocyte populations and T-lymphocyte subsets in head and neck squamous cell carcinomas from patients receiving perilymphatic injections of recombinant interleukin 2. A pathologic and immunophenotypic study. Modern Pathology 1990; 3:702-708.
55. Whiteside TL, Letessier E, Hirabayashi H, Vitolo D, Bryant J, Barnes L, Snyderman C, Johnson JT, Myers E, Herberman RB, Rubin J, Kirkwood JM, Vlock DR. Evidence for local and systemic activation of immune cells by peritumoral injections of interleukin 2 in patients with advanced squamous cell carcinoma of the head and neck. Submitted 1993.
56. Weidmann E, Sacchi M, Plaisance S, Heo DS, Yasumura S, Lin WC, Johnson JT, Herberman RB, Azzarone B, Whiteside TL. Receptors for interleukin 2 on human squamous cell carcinoma cell lines and tumor in situ. Cancer Res 1992; 52:5963-5970.
57. Yasumura S, Lin W-C, Weidmann E, Hebda P, Whiteside TL. Expression of interleukin 2 receptors on human carcinoma cell lines and tumor growth inhibition by interleukin 2. Submitted 1993.
58. Rimoldi D, Salvi S, Hartmann F, Schreyer M, Blum S, Zografos L, Plaisance S, Azzarone B, Carrel S. Expression of IL-2 receptors in human melanoma cells. AntiCancer Res 1993; 13:555-564.
59. Columbo MP, Modesti A, Parmiani G, Forni G. Local cytokine availability elicits tumor rejection and systemic immunity through granulocyte-T lymphocyte cross talk. Cancer Res 1992; 52:4853-4857.
60. Whiteside-Nimick TL. Growth inhibitory effects of cytokines on human head and neck cancer in vitro and in vivo. In: Johnson JT, Didolkar MS., eds.Head and Neck Cancer, Volume III. The Netherlands: Elsevier Science Publishers, 1993: 145-151.
61. Fearon ER, Pardoll DM, Itaya T, Golumbek P, Levitsky HI, Simons JW, Karasuyama H, Vogelstein B, Frost P. Interleukin-2 production by tumor cells bypasses T helper function in the generation of an antitumor response. Cell 1990; 60:397-403.
62. Golumbek PT, Lazenby AJ, Levitsky HI, Jaffee LM, Karasuyama H, Baker M, Pardoll DM. Treatment of established renal cancer by tumor cells engineered to secrete interleukin-4. Science 1991; 254:713-716.
63. Gansbacher B, Zier K, Daniels B, Cronin K, Bannerji R, Gilboa E. Interleukin 2 gene transfer into tumor cells abrogates tumorigenicity and induces protected immunity. J Exp Med 1990; 172:1217-1224.

CHAPTER 8

Adoptive Immunotherapy with TIL

Human solid tumors AIT with antitumor effector cells plus cytokines have been receiving a great deal of attention in recent years. AIT is based upon the premise that an effective cell-mediated immune response can be generated against cancer and that this process can be harnessed and developed into an effective treatment modality. Largely due to efforts of Steven Rosenberg and his collaborators, AIT, first with PHA activated peripheral blood lymphocytes,[1] later with LAK cells,[2,3] and then with TIL, has emerged as a novel and promising approach to treatment of patients with metastatic disease.[4,5] The promise offered by AIT with TIL, and the enthusiasm generated by its application to treatment of patients with metastatic disease unresponsive to conventional therapies have not been tempered by the fact that more than 70% of patients remained unresponsive to AIT or by practical and financial difficulties imposed by this form of therapy. Currently, it remains one of the best characterized and, in some patients with melanoma, effective clinical approaches to immunotherapy of advanced, metastatic cancer.

There are at least three reasons for focusing on TIL as a source of immune antitumor effector cells for AIT of cancer: (a) TIL may be enriched in AuTu-specific CTL; (b) TIL are generally responsive to activation with exogenous IL-2 and expand sufficiently well ex vivo to yield large numbers of cells thought to be necessary for therapy; and (c) in vitro-activated TIL transferred to tumor-bearing hosts appear to localize to the tumor site or its metastases. It has been suggested that these characteristics of TIL, including class I MHC restriction, distinguish them from other types of non-MHC-restricted effector cells used for AIT such as, e.g., LAK cells.[6,7] AIT with TIL is based on solid preclinical evidence obtained in experimental animal models, which indicated that TIL might represent a better source of antitumor effector cells than PBL. TIL were shown to be 50-100 fold more effective than LAK cells in eliminating established pulmonary metastases in a murine sarcoma model after pretreatment with cyclophosphamide and in the presence of exogenous IL-2.[8] Rosenberg and colleagues also reported long-lasting responses in a proportion of patients with metastatic melanoma or RCC treated with TIL/IL-2.[5] These experimental and clinical studies have indicated that AIT with TIL/IL-2 can lead to regression of established or even bulky tumors in tumor-bearing hosts.

More recently, as a result of intensive basic and clinical investigations conducted with TIL obtained from a variety of human solid tumors, some skepticism has developed about effectiveness of AIT with TIL. The frequency of responses in patients with melanoma or RCC treated with TIL/IL-2 has not been unequivocally higher than that obtained with IL-2 alone, LAK cells and IL-2 or more conventional therapies. Although the response rate was 55% in 20 patients with metastatic melanoma, including several who failed previous LAK therapy in an initial report from the NCI,[5] it has been noted that the response rate calculated on the basis of intent to treat (20 additional patients were biopsied for TIL cultures but were not treated due to a rapid disease progression (or inadequate TIL growth) was only 28%.[5,9] This figure was not statistically different from results obtained in LAK/IL-2 studies, where all patients entered could be treated.

Today, it remains unconfirmed that TIL from tumors other than melanoma or RCC can be expanded in vitro and successfully used for AIT. No clinical or laboratory predictors have been identified that correlate with a likelihood of response. Objective evaluation of TIL therapy has been confounded by the lack of well-defined, uniform criteria for culture and administration of TIL. Few clinical trials with TIL/IL-2 have been completed to date, and there exists a great need for additional information about therapeutic efficacy of human TIL. In this chapter, various aspects of AIT with TIL will be covered, and the future of this form of therapy will be critically assessed. In addition, information about the mechanisms which might mediate or influence clinical responses will be discussed.

PREPARATION OF TIL FOR THERAPEUTIC PROTOCOLS

In cancer patients the clinical phase I trials completed to date have indicated that partial and complete responses can occur following systemic AIT with TIL in a proportion of patients who had not responded to conventional therapies.[4,5] However, AIT is not yet a standard therapeutic modality available on a routine basis, and it can only be provided to patients with cancer under the investigational new drug (IND) category following approval by the Food and Drug Administration (FDA) of a cell generation process at a given laboratory. Isolation and culture of TIL for AIT require good laboratory practice, which meets the FDA requirements.

Implementation of these requirements represents a considerable investment of technical effort as well as resources, but, in general, preparation of cells for AIT is within the capabilities of any cell-mediated immunity laboratory willing to adopt the additional measures of quality control and safety which are required for therapeutic products. We and others have recently described a procedure for preparation and culture of human TIL for AIT[10,11] as performed in a clinical laboratory. Currently, cells prepared for AIT represent an IND and can be administered to patients under the guidelines of a clinical protocol only after the IND is filed and approved by the FDA. A laboratory preparing the cells has to document its record in successful product generation and validate the procedures used for the production process. The guidelines for these procedures can be requested from the Division of Cancer Treatment, BRMP, Frederick, MD.

A facility for the production of human cells for AIT should be solely dedicated to this purpose. The laboratory needs to be equipped with a laminar flow hood for tissue culture, CO_2 incubators, centrifuges and other cell-separation equipment, microscopes, water baths and a refrigerator/freezer. It is advisable that only sterile disposable plastics be used for tissue culture and other procedures. While it is not necessary to provide positive pressure or filtered air system for the laboratory, the access to it should be limited, and the personnel requested to wear clean laboratory attire at all times. The laboratory should be supervised by a qualified professional experienced in tissue culture of human cells and cognizant of required quality control and sterility of the product.

All reagents, enzymes and culture media used for TIL preparation must be fresh and sterile. Culture media for TIL expansion are purchased bottled and sterile from a qualified vendor. Human AB serum for use as a medium supplement should be obtained from a licensed blood bank or registered plasmapheresis center or purchased in one large pretested lot from a reliable vendor, who holds a master file with the Center for Biologics Evaluation and Research, FDA. Human serum must be obtained from donors nonreactive for hepatitis, human immunodeficiency virus (HIV) or human lymphotropic virus type 1 (HTLV-1). It must be free of adventitious agents, and pretested for its ability to support growth of effector cells. Serum-free media, e.g., AIM-V, are preferable for culture of TIL because of safety and reduction in cost. Complete culture media prepared by mixing different sterile components must be filtered through a 0.22μm disposable filter prior to use. Choice of antibiotics to be used in culture should be carefully considered: if there are indications for penicillin sensitivity in a patient who is to receive AIT, gentamicin should be used to replace penicillin in culture media. Human recombinant IL-2 preparations or other cytokines, e.g., IL-4 or IL-7, used for activation and/or culture must be approved by the FDA for in vivo use in humans.

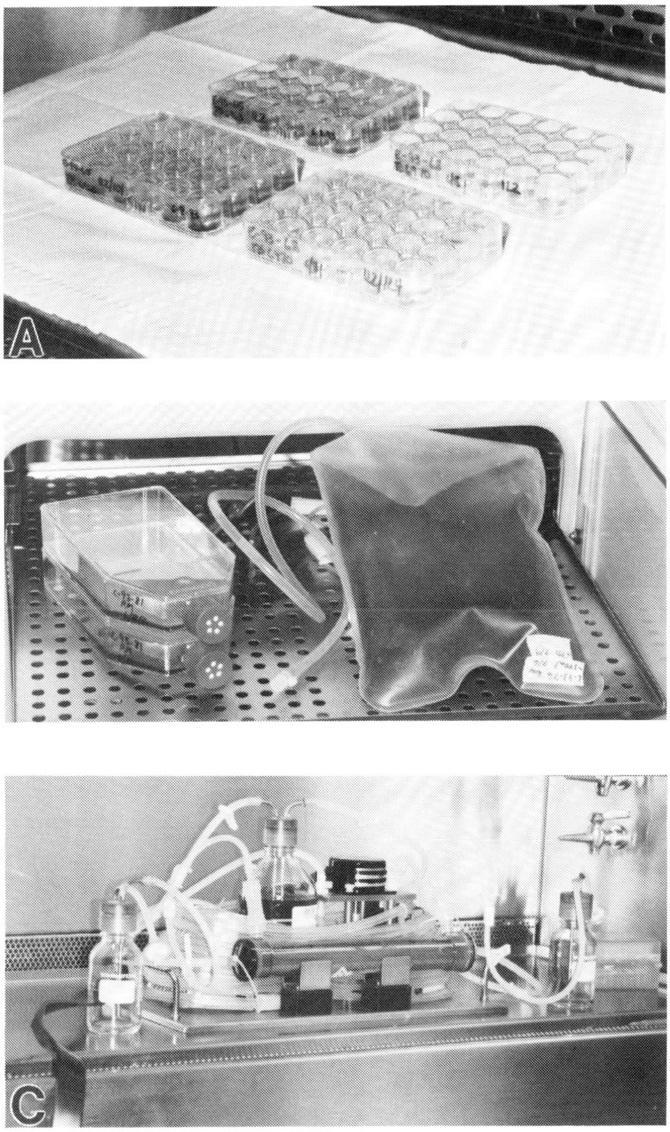

Fig. 1. Culture of human TIL expanding in the presence of IL-2 first in 24-well culture plates (a) then in Fenwal gas permeable plastic bags (b) or in a hollow-fiber device (c). Plates, bags or HFD are placed in a 37°C incubator and cultured under conditions described in the text.

To obtain TIL for AIT, these cells must be first isolated from tumor tissues by mechanical and enzymatic digestion, as described in Chapter 3. For enzymatic digestion, freshly-harvested tumor tissue is first minced in medium into <1 mm^3 pieces with scalpels under sterile conditions. A mixture of collagenase (type V; 0.4 mg/ml) and DNAse (0.2 mg/ml), prepared in advance and filtered through a 0.22 μm-pore-size disposable filter, is used for digestion, which varies in length from 1 to 12h, depending on the tumor. The enzymatic treatment is performed in a trypsinization flask placed on a magnetic stirrer in a 37°C water bath. TIL suspensions are then centrifuged, washed in medium, adjusted to the cell concentration of 0.5 x 10^6/ml and placed in wells of 24-well plates for culture.

Following the initial culture in 24-well plates (Fig. 1a), TIL are transferred to 6-well

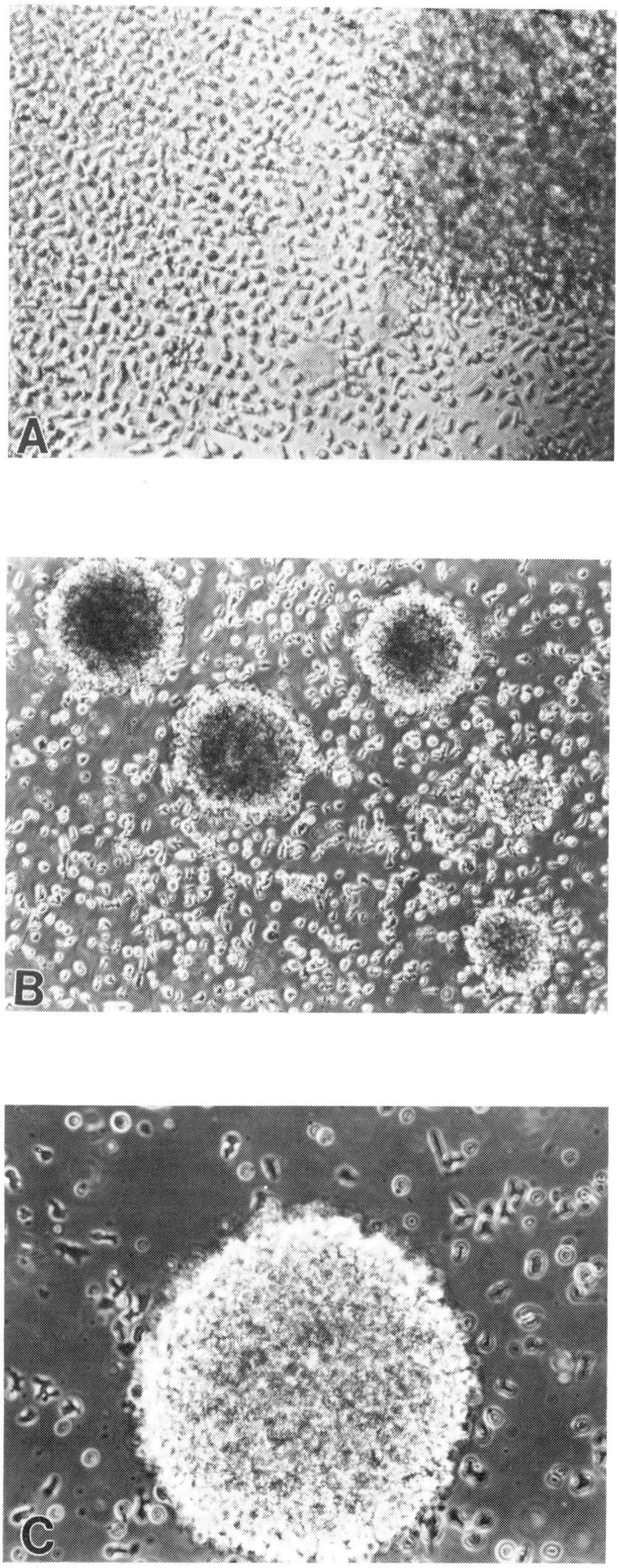

Fig. 2. Growth of human TIL in AIM-V medium containing 6000 IU/ml of IL-2. Initially, the cells expand as a single cell suspension (a). As the cell number increases, aggregates of CD3⁺ T lymphocytes begin to form (b) Mag x 100, and these enlarge to very substantial aggregates floating in the culture medium. Mag x 200.

plates and expanded further until at least 2 x 10^8 cells in the log phase of growth are obtained. At this point, TIL can be transferred to a hollow fiber device (HFD)[12]. The minimum number of TIL for transfer to a HFD is about 2 x 10^8. The best results are obtained when the TIL culture is scaled up gradually, working in wells of culture plates and/or small flasks prior to transferring the cells to bags or automated equipment (Fig. 1). In plates or flasks, TIL grow as nonadherent, free-floating cells which tend to form large aggregates (Fig. 2). Automated cell culture equipment such as HFD reduces opportunities for contamination and makes handling of large cell numbers feasible without a need for extensive incubator space, which is required for bags. Expansion of TIL in hollow fiber cylinders can be excellent, as indicated in Figure 3. To recover TIL from HFD, it is necessary to carefully wash extrafiber space with medium, using gentle tapping of the cartridge to dislodge the cells growing along the fibers. Viability and cell concentration should be monitored at regular intervals during culture, and all manipulations, sampling, and media or IL-2 additions must be done under sterile conditions. Records of cell numbers and feeding schedules have to be scrupulously maintained.

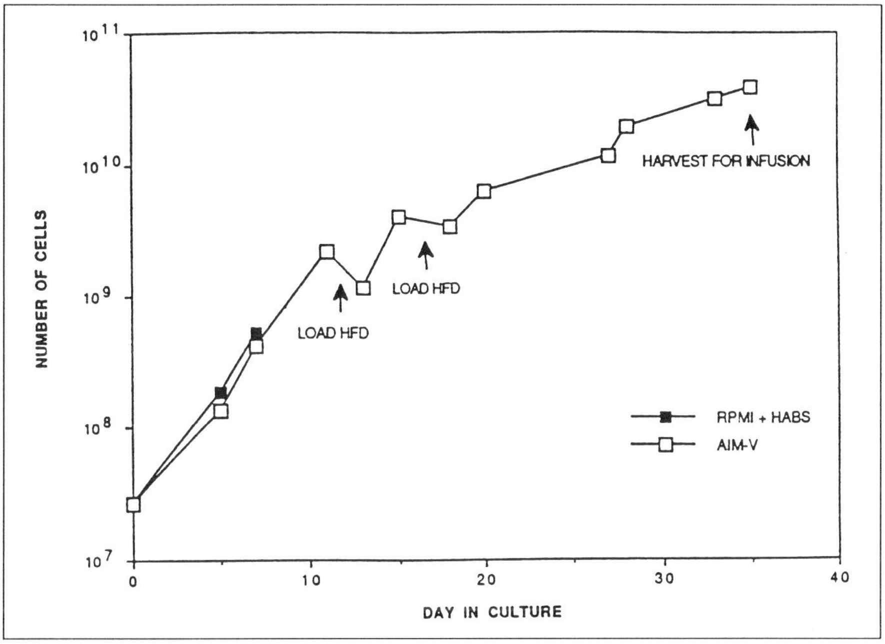

Fig. 3. Growth curve for human TIL in AIM-V medium and IL-2 (6,000 IU/ml) in a hollow fiber device (HFD). TIL were obtained from a patient with malignant melanoma and were initially cultured in wells of 24-well plates in either AIM-V or RPMI plus human AB serum and IL-2. The automatic device was loaded with TIL twice, as indicated, to assure a complete transfer of all TIL expanded in plates. TIL were cultured in HFD for about 20 days.

Cell cultures being prepared for therapy should be continuously supervised by qualified personnel. Detailed standard operating procedures should be maintained in the laboratory and updated by a supervisor at regular intervals. If cultures from more than one patient are prepared, cross-contamination must be avoided by strictly implementing the following rules: only cells of one patient are handled at any given time, culture vessels are clearly labeled and dated, cells obtained from each patient are incubated in different chambers of an CO_2 incubator, only disposable plastics are employed, decontamination of incubators and hood spaces is implemented in-between handling of cells of different patients. Quality control procedures should be in effect at all times during cell culture to qualify reagents, media, plasticware as well as processing and handling of cells.

Prior to AIT, each lot of activated or cultured cells has to be tested for sterility, yield and viability, purity, and antitumor activity. Forty-eight hours prior to harvesting of cells, a sample of culture representing about 5% of the total volume is removed from each cell lot for bacteriologic cultures and mycoplasma testing. Sterility testing is repeated on the day of therapy. Gram stain is also performed at that time. Absence of tumor or tissue cells in the final product must be documented microscopically on H & E-stained smears. Harvested cells are counted in the presence of a trypan blue dye to confirm that viability is >90%. Flow cytometry is performed on an aliquot of the harvested culture to determine the phenotype of cultured TIL. Measurements of cytotoxicity of cultured cells in four hour ^{51}Cr-release assays against AuTu or allogeneic tumor cell targets at different effector to target (E:T) ratios should be performed on another harvested aliquot. Criteria need to be established by each laboratory regarding acceptance vs. rejection of cellular products prepared for AIT. Cellular products must be sterile and free of adventitious agents, safe as well as phenotypically and functionally defined.

This type of validation for TIL to be used for AIT is a requirement, and laboratories preparing this cellular product must be able to provide written records to document compliance.

More recently, TIL transduced with the NeoR gene or TNF-α gene have been used for AIT.[13] The NeoR gene serves as a marker for TIL infused to a patient in order to follow their localization to the tumor, and the TNF-α gene is expected to improve therapeutic efficacy of TIL.[13] Transductions of TIL with human genes delivered by retroviral vectors and expansion of transduced cells for AIT should be performed in a laboratory specifically designated for this purpose and away from cultures of other cellular products prepared for therapy. Retroviral vectors used for therapeutic purposes contain a defective, genetically-modified retrovirus, such as Moloney murine leukemia virus (LNL6), which is unable to replicate. Therapy with genetically-modified TIL cannot be performed without approval from the Recombinant DNA Advisory Committee (RAC) of the NIH, Washington, DC. To obtain such an approval, safety of the viral vectors must be first documented. The titer of viral SN used for transduction should be sufficiently high to assure satisfactory transduction efficiency during a reasonably short period of their incubation (e.g., two hours) with TIL. The efficiency of transduction is determined by PCR for the NeoR gene insertion and by neomycin phosphotransferase (NPT) dot blot analysis for function. Genetically-modified TIL are cultured without selection, mainly to avoid a loss of cells during the selection procedure in the presence of the neomycin analogue, G418. As a consequence of omitting selection, only a portion of total TIL infused to a patient will be carrying the transduced gene. Since the rationale for this approach is to mark TIL with the NeoR gene, and since the PCR-based read-out procedure is very sensitive, the lack of selection of transfectants appears to be justifiable in this case.

Before genetically-modified TIL can be infused to patients, it is necessary to ascertain that the cultured harvested cells contain the NeoR gene. This is done by PCR, using sets of specific primers. In addition, TIL are assayed for the expression of the NeoR gene in a neomycin phosphotransferase assay. Safety testing of each TIL preparation involves the S^+/L^- assay after 3T3 amplification to show that no viral particles capable of replicating are present in TIL cultures and the "autonomous growth" assay (see Fig. 4) to demonstrate that gene-modified TIL are unable to grow autonomously in the absence of IL-2.

To help the reader understand the process of TIL expansion, transduction and preparation of the final product for AIT, Tables 1 and 2 are provided. The data shown in these two tables were obtained in our laboratory, using TIL obtained from two patients with melanoma who were recently treated with gene-modified TIL by Dr. Michael T. Lotze at the Pittsburgh Cancer Institute. In preparing these TIL cultures for therapy, we cultured cells transduced with the NeoR gene separately from the main culture growing in a HFD. Growth of both transduced as well as nontransduced TIL was monitored, and, as shown in Figure 5, transduced TIL expanded comparably to their nontransduced counterpart. Table 1 shows the numbers of TIL generated at various stages of culture, and Table 2 summarizes phenotypic and functional characteristics of the cells which were used for therapy and gives the results of other assays performed with the cultures prior to therapeutic infusions. It is interesting to note that the Patient 1 was treated mainly with activated $CD4^+$ T cells, while the Patient 2 received a mixture of $CD8^+$ and $CD4^+$ TIL. In vitro AuTu cytotoxicity of both TIL preparations was low, although it seemed to be largely selective for melanoma targets, as these TIL did not lyse K562 or Daudi targets to any substantial degree (Table 2).

IMMUNOTHERAPY WITH TIL/IL-2 VS IL-2 ALONE

Many clinical trials have been performed using adoptively transferred LAK cells and IL-2.[2,3,14-19] This combination of biologic agents has been shown to be most effective in patients with melanoma or RCC.[17] However, it has been observed that IL-2 alone can generate similar response rates in patients with melanoma, implying that LAK cells do

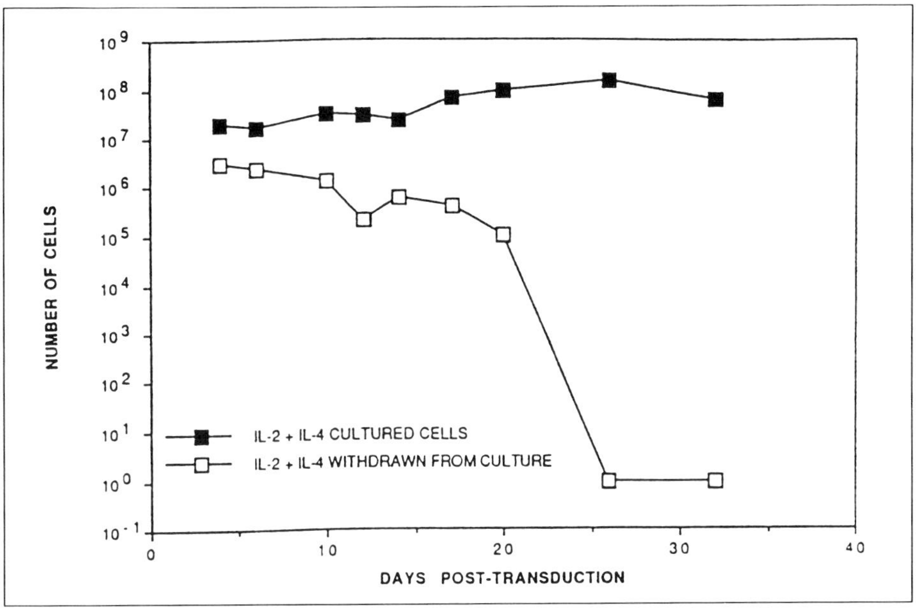

Fig. 4. TIL transduced with the NeoR gene and cultured in the presence of IL-2 (6,000 IU/ml) and IL-4 (1,000 U/ml) were tested for the ability to proliferate in the absence of exogenous IL-2 and IL-4. When the cytokines were eliminated, the culture ceased to proliferate, indicating that the transduced TIL were unable to proliferate autonomously.

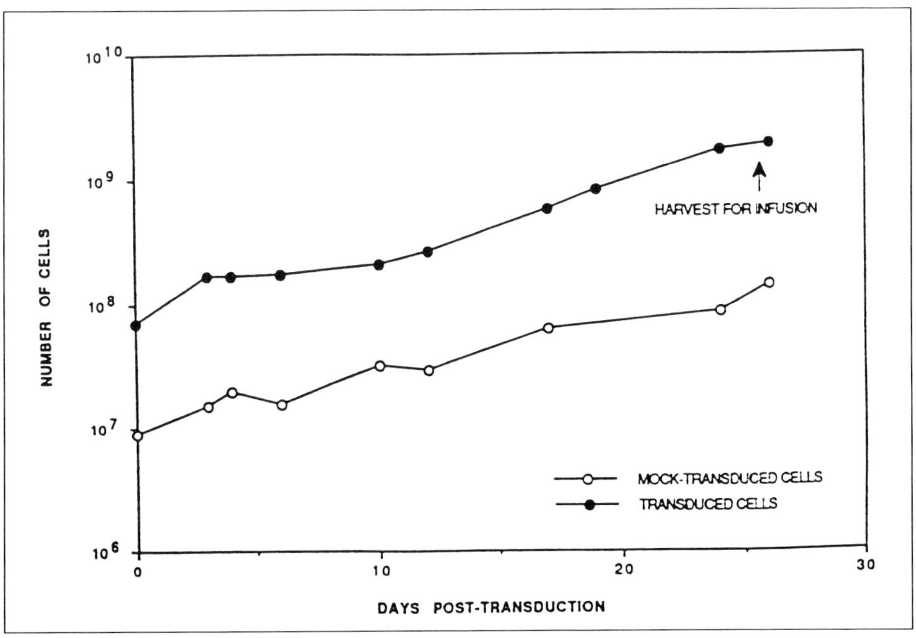

Fig. 5. Growth curves for TIL transduced with the NeoR gene and for the mock-transduced TIL. TIL were obtained from a patient with melanoma and cultured in the presence of IL-2 and IL-4 in AIM-V medium. A portion of the culture was transduced with the NeoR gene, and the transduced TIL cultured in parallel with mock-transduced TIL. Note that the slopes of both growth curves are nearly the same.

Table 1. Culture and gene transfection with the neomycin resistance gene of TIL obtained from patients with metastatic melanoma[a]

	Patient 1	Patient 2
SPECIMEN	Cutaneous nodule	Skin lesion
Weight (g)	8.0	4.8
Cells in suspension (No.)[b]	1×10^8	8.0×10^7
Viability (%)	80	90
INITIAL CULTURE		
Total cell (No.)	1×10^8	1×10^8
Lymphocytes (No.)	2.3×10^7	5.4×10^7
Lymphocytes (%)	25	50
Total cells at time of transfer to HFD (No.)	9.4×10^8	1.1×10^9
TRANSFECTION		
Day in culture	17	8
MOI	2	2
Cells transfected (No.)	8×10^7	7×10^7
Transfected cells recovered (No.)	3.4×10^9	2.0×10^9
HARVEST FOR INFUSION		
Day in culture	46	34
Total cells (No.)	3.4×10^{10}	9.9×10^{10}
Transduced cells (%)	10	2
Expansion fold	35	31

[a] Suspensions of TIL and tumor cells were obtained by enzymatic digestion of tumor tissues and initially cultured in 24-well plates. A part of the TIL culture was reserved for transfection of TIL with the NeoR gene by incubating TIL with G_1Na viral supernatants (multiplicity of infection, MOI, of 2) for two hours. The remaining TIL expanded in plates were then transferred to a hollow fiber device (HFD) and cultured until the time of harvest. At the time of harvest for therapy, transfected TIL were combined with nontransfected TIL recovered from the HFD, and all cells were intravenously infused to the patient.

[b] Cells in tumor suspension contained tumor cells and MNC.

not add to the efficacy of this treatment.[19] Rosenberg and colleagues have compared response and survival rates in 181 patients, 97 with RCC and 54 with melanoma, treated with high-dose IL-2 alone or with LAK/IL-2.[20] The patients were followed for 63.2 months (median). Among the 90 patients who were randomly assigned to receive LAK/IL-2, 24 (27%) had objective regressions of metastatic disease, and among the 91 patients who received IL-2, 16 (18%) had objective cancer regression. There were 10 complete responses (CR) among the 85 evaluable patients treated with LAK/IL-2, compared with 4 among 79 who received IL-2 alone. There were 14 and 12 partial responses (PR), respectively. Seven patients are in complete response 50–66 months after therapy. The data suggested a trend toward increased survival in patients with melanoma treated with LAK/IL-2 but not in patients with RCC. Factors that might be associated with response and thus, be of predictive value in identifying and selecting patients most likely to respond to this therapy, were not identified in this trial. The results were not as encouraging as originally expected, considering the extent of effort and cost of therapy.

Table 2. Characteristics of TIL cultured for therapy in a hollow fiber device and infused to patients[a]

		Patient 1	Patient 2
PHENOTYPE:	$CD3^+$	97	98
(% positive)	$CD4^+$	80	58
	$CD8^+$	17	39
	$CD56^+$	1	1
	$CD25^+$	56	15
	$HLA\text{-}DR^+$	67	93
CYTOTOXICITY:	K562	2	14
($LU_{20}/10^7$ cells)	Daudi	8	9
	FEM-X	8	75
	AuTu	45	61
STERILITY		Yes	Yes
CYTOLOGY		No tumor cells	No tumor cells
AUTONOMOUS GROWTH		None	None
HELPER VIRUS		None	None
ENDOTOXIN		<0.08 EU	<0.08 EU

[a] TIL were obtained from two patients with melanoma and cultured as indicated in Table 3. The phenotype of cultured TIL was determined by two-color flow cytometry, and cytotoxicity of TIL against the tumor cell targets listed was tested in 4h ^{51}Cr-release assays. All tests were performed immediately prior to TIL infusion to patients. EU = endotoxin units. FEM-X is an allogeneic melanoma cell line.

Nevertheless, it should be recognized that 27% of patients with metastatic disease unresponsive to conventional therapy have been able to achieve responses with AIT and that some of these responses have been long lasting.[20]

Strategies to improve antitumor activity of adoptively transferred cells are being actively investigated, and among these strategies, therapy with tumor-specific cytotoxic T cells has been championed by Steven Rosenberg at the Surgery Branch, NCI.[4,5] Based on extensive in vitro preclinical studies, Rosenberg and colleagues have suggested that TIL are a source of tumor-specific cytotoxic T cells, at least in patients with melanoma.[21,22] Although this remains one of the most controversial aspects of TIL therapy, in some cases, TIL generated from melanoma have been identified as class I MHC-restricted $CD3^+CD8^+$ T cells able to recognize and kill AuTu.[21,22] In most instances, however, therapeutic TIL cultures are mixtures of various proportions of $CD4^+$ and $CD8^+$ T lymphocytes, most of which are MHC-unrestricted. In contrast, LAK cells are predominantly $CD3^-$ $CD56^+$ and $CD16^+$ NK cells, although T cells may account for a substantial proportion of cultured LAK cells.[23] The rationale of AIT with TIL is based on the hypothesis that AuTu-specific cytolytic T cells are more effective in mediating antitumor responses than non-MHC-restricted effector cells.[24] Systemic administration of TIL and of IL-2 at doses which have varied from high to moderate (e.g., from 30 x 10^6 IU/kg to 30 x 10^5 IU/kg as a cumulative dose) is based on a notion that IL-2 is necessary to sustain in vivo effectiveness of transferred TIL. In fact, high doses of systemic IL-2 given to patients in conjunction with effector cells appeared to be responsible for considerable toxicity that is associated with this form of therapy (see below). As more experience with IL-2-based immunotherapy accumulates, it appears that high doses of IL-2 may not be essential or even advisable to support transferred TIL, because favorable response rates are being reported with effector cells plus low doses of IL-2.[25] In place of early practice of using high doses of IL-2 as a bolus, modifications including continuous IL-2 delivery or decrescendo IL-2 therapy[26] have resulted in diminished and tolerable IL-2-related toxicities.

Another concern about TIL protocols is related to the perception that IL-2 alone may be more or equally as effective as TIL/IL-2. However, careful examination of clinical responses obtained with TIL and IL-2 in patients who had previously failed to respond to IL-2 alone indicated that the addition of TIL resulted in partial and complete responses in a considerable proportion of these individuals (M.T. Lotze, personal communication). Similarly, experiments performed by Dr. James Mule at the Surgery Branch, NCI, indicated that effector cells plus IL-2 were consistently and significantly more effective than IL-2 alone against pulmonary metastases in a wide variety of histologic types of tumors in mice.[27] It thus appears that utilization of adoptively transferred cells in addition to cytokines remains a promising therapeutic option. While both generation and therapy with TIL have generally included IL-2, attempts are being made to use a combination of IL-2 plus IL-4[28] or IL-2 plus IL-7[29] in order to improve the quality of the product as well as clinical efficacy of therapy with TIL.

REVIEW OF CLINICAL TRIALS WITH TIL PLUS IL-2

Table 3 provides a summary of currently available results of clinical trials with TIL/IL-2 in patients with cancer.[4,5,30-34] The total of eight clinical trials with TIL, of which three were performed at the Surgery Branch, NCI, have been completed and the results published. This represents a total of 153 patients, mostly with melanoma, who have received TIL/IL-2 therapy. Clinical responses (either CR or PR) were reported in 36 of these patients for the response rate of 24%.

Table 3. Currently available results of clinical trials with TIL/IL-2 in patients with cancer

All tumor types Number E/R	%R	Melanoma	RCC	Colon	Lung	Breast	Year	Reference
		Number of patients E/R						
12/3	25	6/1	4/1PR	1/0	-	1/1PR	1988	Topalian (4)
20/11	55	20/11 (1 CR)	-	-	-	-	1988	Rosenberg (5)
28/5	18	13/3	7/2PR	-	8/0	-	1989	Kradin (30)
5/2[a]	40	5/2 (1 CR)	-	-	-	-	1990	Rosenberg (13)
40/5	13	20/4 (1 CR)	Other tumors:			20/1[b]	1991	Oldham (32)
21/5	24	21/5 (1 CR)	-	-	-	-	1991	Dillman (33)
18/0	0	-	18/0	-	-	-	1991	Bukowski (31)
9/5	55	9/5 (1 CR)	-	-	-	-	1992	Rivoltini (34)

Abbreviations: R = responding patients with partial (PR) or complete (CR) responses; E = the number of patients treated with TIL/IL-2 who were evaluable for response.

[a] TIL were transduced with the NeoR gene

[b] Included were patients with RCC, colon carcinoma and lymphoma

Nearly all of the patients treated with TIL had either metastatic melanoma or RCC, and the effectiveness of TIL therapy in a broader array of tumors has not been determined. For 94 patients with melanoma treated with TIL/IL-2, the response rate was 33%. This response rate does not appear to be different from results obtained in LAK/IL-2 studies.[20] In the phase I clinical trial with TIL/IL-2 performed in 18 patients with RCC by Bukowski et al at the Cleveland Clinic, no objective clinical responses were observed.[31] The lack of efficacy of AIT with TIL/IL-2 noted in this trial raises a number of questions regarding the future application of AIT in patients with RCC. Fortunately, this trial was meticulously performed and the patients were carefully monitored for a variety of immunologic parameters so that the observed lack of efficacy could be related to several specific factors. These included the heterogeneity of the cultured TIL in terms of their phenotypic and functional characteristics and the absence of specific AuTu cytotoxicity of cultured TIL. In most cases, these TIL displayed non-MHC-restricted cytotoxicity which was mediated by $CD56^+$ effector cells. Thus, in contrast to melanoma, where specific MHC-restricted CTL derived from tumor can be obtained and cultured for therapy with some consistency, AuTu-specific CTL from RCC appear to be either infrequent among TIL or their culture is particularly difficult.[31]

Based on the results of a limited number of phase I clinical trials performed to date and listed in Table 3, objective evaluation of TIL/IL-2 therapy cannot be made at this time. The results of the trials that have been completed to date are difficult to compare because of the following differences: (a) schedules for TIL/IL-2 administration varied greatly between the trials; (b) therapy with cyclophosphamide was included in some trials but not in others; (c) tremendous variations were observed between patients in TIL growth and the degree of activation. In fact, inability to culture TIL from some patients or to generate sufficient numbers of TIL for therapy prevented their entry on the protocol after several weeks of expansion; (d) it remains unclear whether patients who responded to TIL therapy were treated with TIL populations enriched in $CD8^+$ or $CD4^+$ T cells or whether the transferred TIL were selectively able to kill AuTu; (e) conditions for culture and expansion of TIL varied from one laboratory to another; (f) responses to therapy have not been correlated to changes in the immune function of patients treated with TIL/IL-2; (g) duration of responses has not been clearly specified, and it might be too early to evaluate survival in these relatively recent clinical trials. It seems obvious, that for TIL therapy to be administered successfully, it will be necessary to solve a number of problems, including the recovery of TIL from tumor biopsy, ability to propagate them in vitro and to generate AuTu-specific T cells as well as the availability of AuTu for in vitro assays.

Ex vivo expansion of TIL is only possible in a fraction of patients with cancer. In many cases and for various reasons, tumors obtained from surgery yield few TIL. TIL obtained from metastatic tumors fail to proliferate ex vivo in some cases. Overall, from 30 to 50% of patients considered for TIL therapy may not be treated because of one of the above limitations.[33,34] Thus, while the selection of patients likely to benefit from AIT is important, it is necessary to admit that TIL therapy may not be feasible in many of those who are eligible for AIT. In the absence of a reliable in vitro correlate(s) of clinical response, it is impossible to predict at present which patients are likely to benefit from therapy with TIL.

The toxicities associated with TIL/IL-2 administration and reported in the trials performed to date have mostly reflected the dose and schedule of IL-2 utilized. Fever and/or chills are generally the only toxic effects associated with intravenous TIL infusion. In the recent phase I trial in Cleveland,[31] patients with RCC were treated with TIL and escalating doses of IL-2 (0, 3, 4.5 x 10^6 U/m^2) on days 1 to 5 and 8 to 12. Dose limiting toxicity was pulmonary, and the MTD of IL-2 was 3 x 10^6 U/m^2. Side effects of IL-2-based therapies include malaise, nausea and vomiting, diarrhea, capillary leak syndrome, hypotension, oliguria, weight gain and pulmonary dysfunction.[35,36] IL-2 therapy has also been associated with significant cardiorespiratory and hemodynamic changes similar to those seen in patients with septic shock. Rosenberg and colleagues have focused attention on physiologic and hemodynamic changes associated with administration of TIL.[37] They monitored patients receiving TIL infusions prior to administration of systemic IL-2. A mean of 10 x 10^{10} TIL (range 2-20 x 10^{10}) were infused to 22 patients. Two hours following infusion, the patients developed tachycardia, increased cardiac index, decreased vascular resistance and increased pulmonary diastolic pressure. No correlation was observed between release of TNF-α, IFN-γ or GM-CSF in vitro by TIL and hemodynamic effects following administration of these TIL to patients. Thus, systemic infusion of TIL alone was associated with hemodynamic changes similar to those noted with IL-2 therapy.[37] These results are important, because they emphasize a need for caution during TIL infusions, when general tendency has been to consider such infusions as harmless relative to infusions of IL-2.

GENERATION OF AUTOTUMOR-SPECIFIC TIL FOR THERAPY

The issue of TIL preparation for therapy and cost associated with it has been one aspect of this form of therapy that deserves further attention and where improvements are needed. As used by Rosenberg's group, this therapy calls for administration of 10^{10}-10^{11} TIL and, therefore, requires in vitro expansion of TIL for four to eight weeks depending on the initial cell input.[4,5] Several independent groups have now acquired experience in culturing TIL on a large scale for therapy.[30-34] Although the feasibility of a large-scale TIL culture for therapy has been sufficiently established,[10-12] at least for TIL from melanoma and RCC, optimal conditions for expansion of AuTu-specific T cells remain to be determined. Also, it remains unconfirmed that TIL from other solid tumors can be similarly expanded, and, of course, not all TIL, especially those obtained from metastatic tumors, are able to grow in vitro.[23,38]

Generation of AuTu-specific CTL from TIL requires in vitro selection in the presence of irradiated AuTu or appropriately presented synthetic peptides. While a variety of procedures have been used for in vitro selection of $CD3^+CD8^+$ T cells, including highly-successful separation on anti-CD8 monoclonal antibody-covered surfaces,[39,40] selective expansion of AuTu specific CTL has been much more difficult. To a large extent, the difficulty is associated with the usual paucity of AuTu cells for in vitro activation or with the lack of appropriate synthetic peptides for in vitro sensitization of expanding TIL. There is also uncertainty about restricting therapeutically-administered cells to those with CD8 phenotype. It is possible that $CD4^+$ cells are necessary for optimal in vivo antitumor activities of $CD8^+$ T cells. In the past, patients who have responded to IL-2 therapy, were often treated with mixed lymphocyte populations containing both $CD8^+$ and $CD4^+$ T cells.[4,5,30-34] Still another unanswered question concerns AuTu reactivity of ex vivo activated TIL. It has been claimed recently that the ability to lyse AuTu in vitro is the best correlate of their clinical effectiveness.[41] However, this observation remains unconfirmed, and criteria for the clinically most effective TIL preparation remain to be defined. Although technology exists for massive expansion of TIL in, e.g., HFDs,[12] guidelines for the quality or quantity of the final product to be used therapeutically have not been formulated and are not available.

With respect to clinical or laboratory predictors of response, Marincola and colleagues examined the possibility that HLA phenotype of a patient may be an important correlate of response to IL-2-based therapies.[42] It is reasonable to hypothesize that different HLA haplotypes could differ in the ability to present tumor-specific endogenous antigens, so that patients with various HLA phenotypes may tend to respond differently to therapy aimed at improving AuTu responses. The study, which included 146 patients with melanoma, suggested that some class I HLA specificities (e.g., HLA-A1) may indeed predict for a greater likelihood of response to IL-2-based therapy.[42] For patients receiving TIL therapy, responders also had increased frequency of HLA-A19. In addition, the authors observed significant association between HLA-DR4 haplotype and decreased tolerance to IL-2 among the patients who received TIL/IL-2. This retrospective analysis showed that a significant correlation existed between class II HLA phenotype and IL-2-induced toxicity in patients with melanoma treated with TIL/IL-2 and that certain class I HLA specificities correlated with the likelihood of response.[42]

The expense of TIL therapy, currently estimated at $10,000-15,000 per patient, is largely due to long-term in vitro culture (from four to eight weeks) which is necessary to generate cell numbers sufficient for therapy. In vitro strategies aimed at facilitating outgrowth of AuTu-specific TIL would considerably increase the complexity and cost of the preparation of a therapeutic cellular product. Against these expenditures in cost and effort for culturing of TIL, it is necessary to balance significant gains already achieved in: (a) the clinical arena, in respect to evaluation of side effects of TIL therapy, which seem to be mostly, but not entirely,[37] attributable to concurrently administered cytokines or confirmation of feasibility, safety and efficacy of TIL immunotherapy, which has resulted in complete responses in a small number of patients with metastatic disease who did not respond to conventional therapy; (b) basic scientific investigations of biologic properties of human TIL, their antitumor properties, their movement through vasculature into tumors or the mechanisms involved in elimination by TIL of tumor metastases; and (c) increased awareness of clinicians and the scientific community of a possible new approach to cancer therapy with the potential for developing into a major therapeutic modality in the future.

LOCALIZATION OF TIL TO TUMORS

An important question in respect to immunotherapy with TIL is whether these cells infused systemically to patients with cancer are able to preferentially localize to tumor or its metastases. The antitumor mechanisms mediated by in vitro activated and systemically administered TIL are presently unknown. If it is assumed that these TIL-T eliminate AuTu via their cytolytic activity, then localization of in vitro activated TIL in sufficient numbers to the tumor or its metastases becomes a key requirement for successful therapy. Localization of human TIL labeled with ^{111}In to tumor was demonstrated by Fisher et al[43] and Griffith et al[44] for patients with melanoma. Tumor localization of label was seen in 13/18 patients, but only a small percentage of total label (0.0049%/g of tissue) was found in the tumor. Nevertheless, this was ten-fold greater than the label found in normal adjacent skin. In some of these patients, ^{111}In-labeled fresh A-PBL were infused, and the label uptake was determined to be 0.001%/g of tissue in the tumor and 0.004%/g of tissue in normal skin.[44] These experiments suggested that human TIL preferentially localized to the tumor, although a very small proportion of total TIL administered which localized to the tumor might not be sufficient to mediate tumor cell lysis. A while ago, Mukherji and colleagues, compared human ^{111}In-labeled antimelanoma CTL with LAK cells for the ability to target melanoma lesions and found the former significantly more effective.[45] However, it remains unclear how many TIL-T are needed to induce tumor regression in vivo. Indeed, if mechanisms other than direct cytotoxicity are responsible for antitumor effects, i.e., vascular events resulting from endothelial cell-TIL interactions[46] or a cytokine cascade leading to intense local inflammation,[47] then very few TIL might be necessary to bring about tumor regression. Also, the fact that therapeutic transfer of $CD4^+$ TIL has resulted in clinical responses[33,48] might suggest involvement of mechanisms other than direct AuTu cytotoxicity in antitumor responses mediated by immune effector cells. The length of time during which infused TIL remain at the tumor site may also be important, as well as the ability of these TIL to divide in situ.[49,50] Human TIL containing a transduced NeoR gene and administered to patients with melanoma persisted in the circulation for three to eight weeks and were recovered from tumor biopsies in three of five patients in a recent series of experiments in Rosenberg's laboratory.[13] Studies in mice bearing pulmonary metastases of methylcholanthrene-induced sarcoma showed that adoptively transferred TIL persisted at tumor sites for up to 115 days and functioned as memory T cells.[49,50] These studies have provided support for a notion that systemically-delivered TIL which localize to the tumor might persist there as functional cells for prolonged periods of time.

Recent improvements in in vivo tracking of TIL and other effector cells have been obtained through the use of lipophilic compounds which become stably incorporated into the lipid bilayer of cellular membranes.[51] These tracking compounds, when used at suitably adjusted concentrations, do not interfere with cellular functions of lymphocytes and do not impair their viability or ability to localize to tissues, including tumors.[51] Most important, labeling of murine TIL with these compounds does not seem to interfere with their ability to mediate in vivo regression of established pulmonary metastases.[52] Using TIL labeled with fluoresceinated PKH26 or radio-iodinated PHK95, Wallace et al were unable to confirm earlier data that TIL selectively accumulate or proliferate at the tumor site.[52] These recent results are at odds with apparent therapeutic efficacy of TIL observed in the same tumor-bearing animals. Furthermore, they leave unanswered the question about the nature of antitumor mechanism that may be responsible for tumor regression following TIL therapy.

The possibility of genetic "marking" of TIL offers an opportunity for solving unanswered questions in respect to localization of these cells to the tumor site. Human TIL transduced with the LNL6 vector containing the NeoR gene have been identified in tumor biopsies and PBL repeatedly for several weeks following TIL infusion into patients with cancer.[13] However, experiments demonstrating the presence of genetically-marked TIL in tumor biopsies have been limited, and additional studies are needed to confirm the initial results reported by Rosenberg's group.[13] Also, it remains unproven that TIL preferentially localize to the tumor relative to another type of autologous effector cell, e.g., IL-2-activated PBL. The possibility now exists of using two different retroviral vectors for in vivo trafficking studies, in which TIL and "control" A-PBL could be genetically labeled, each with a different gene, and simultaneously infused to cancer patients. The relative ratios of these genetically-marked lymphocyte populations in tumor, blood and normal tissue biopsies could then be compared. A clinical protocol incorporating this strategy is now in progress at UCLA Medical Center in Los Angeles, CA.

AIT WITH GENETICALLY-MODIFIED TIL

To optimize efficacy of AIT with human TIL and to gain insights into their in vivo distribution and survival, a novel strategy of inserting a "marker" gene into cultured TIL was introduced by Rosenberg et al in 1990.[13] Retrovirus-mediated gene transduction was used to introduce the NeoR gene into TIL before their infusion into patients. In theory, the TIL marked with the NeoR gene and their offspring can be identified in patients' circulation or tissues for as long as they survive.[13] To detect marked TIL in patients' blood or tissue, Rosenberg et al used PCR which is able to identify one labeled cell among 10^4 to 10×10^5 unmodified cells. Since a viral vector was used for transduction (LNL6, a derivative of Moloney leukemia virus in which *gag*, *pol* and *env* genes have been removed), careful consideration was given to the potential hazards of using a retrovirus to transfer the NeoR marker gene into TIL. Although the retrovirus was modified and could not replicate, it was necessary to perform safety testing and demonstrate that no viral particles capable of replicating were present in the TIL preparations used for therapy. To this end, the transduced TIL were tested in the S^+L^- assays after 3T3 amplification for the presence of viral envelope genes and of reverse transcriptase.[13] The assays are capable of detecting a single viral particle capable of replication per ml of TIL suspension. Furthermore, TIL were examined for the ability to express the NeoR gene, by testing for the presence of the bacterial gene product, neomycin phosphotransferase. The TIL were also tested for the ability to grow autonomously in the absence of IL-2 and found to be unable to survive in its absence.

Rosenberg and collaborators treated five patients with advanced melanoma using AIT with genetically "marked" TIL, which in four out of five cases grew successfully in high concentrations of G418, a neomycin analogue otherwise toxic to eukaryotic cells.[13] The study demonstrated that patients with cancer could be safely treated with genetically-modified TIL and that the small number of transduced cells persisted in the circulation of all patients for at least three weeks and of two patients for two months and could be detected using PCR. The NeoR gene-transduced cells were detected and could be recovered from tumor deposits in three out of five patients between six days and two months after TIL transfer. Most important, no ill effects of the gene transduction were detected in the patients, and antitumor effects of TIL/IL-2 therapy were seen in three patients.[13] This first clinical study with retrovirus-modified TIL represents a milestone in AIT of cancer. By demonstrating safety, feasibility and efficacy of this approach, Rosenberg's study introduces a promising new option of gene therapy into the clinical arena. For example, Rosenberg and other investigators are hoping to improve efficacy of AIT with TIL by inserting other genes into these cells, such as TNF-α, IFN-α or IL-2.

CRITERIA FOR THERAPY WITH TIL

The optimal use of TIL in cancer therapy requires that a set of criteria be established to assure uniformity and guide various centers engaged in preparation and administration of TIL to patients. There appears to be a need for uniform guidelines in respect to media, cytokines, feeding schedules, phenotypic and functional characteristics of the cellular product, numbers of cells needed for infusion and controls necessary for quality, safety and sterility of the product. Culture conditions and, especially doses and mixtures of cytokines used may be important variables influencing the nature of cultured TIL. In terms of antitumor function of cultured TIL, a recent report has suggested that clinical response might significantly correlate ($p<0.005$) with the ability of cultured TIL to lyse AuTu in vitro.[41] If this observation could be extended to TIL from tumors other than melanoma and confirmed, it would provide a strong argument for therapy with TIL-T cultured under conditions selecting for outgrowth of AuTu-specific effectors. In respect to potential positive correlation between AuTu-cell killing activity of effectors and prognosis in patients with cancer in general, a recent report by Uchida et al[53] deserves attention. Fifty patients with primary localized lung cancer were tested at the time of surgery for ability of their PBL to kill AuTu cells.[54] Most patients (85%) whose PBL were effective in vitro against AuTu remained alive and were tumor-free five years after curative surgery, while all patients whose PBL showed no AuTu-killing activity relapsed within 18 months of surgery and died within 42 months. These data indicated that AuTu killing ability of PBL was an important predictive factor for survival.[53,54] This type of analysis has not been applied to TIL, but should AuTu-killing by fresh or cultured TIL prove to be an equally significant prognostic parameter for survival, then both a rationale for therapy with TIL-T and a choice of cancer patients most likely to benefit from such therapy might be strengthened.

Guidelines are needed not only for optimal generation of TIL for therapy but also for uniformity in the administration of TIL/IL-2. At present, therapeutic results obtained at different sites cannot be compared because of differences in the use of various schedules of TIL/IL-2 administration, different doses of cyclophosphamide employed, and various numbers of cells and doses of IL-2 infused. Clearly, this situation is counterproductive to the overall effort of establishing AIT as another therapeutic modality for cancer.

FUTURE POTENTIAL AND LIMITATIONS OF TIL FOR CANCER THERAPY

Much has been learned about human TIL in situ and in culture in recent years, and several major points of encouragement have been identified. For example, finding of AuTu-reactive T cells among TIL with some frequency and partial or complete regression of some tumors in response to adoptive immunotherapy with TIL, despite the presence of advanced disease and still very imperfect therapeutic approach, indicate that therapeutic potential of TIL should be explored further. Limited knowledge of TIL biology, of interactions between TIL and tumor cells or TIL and vascular endothelium, and of the ability of TIL to localize to the tumor obviously hampers the development of better therapeutic approaches with TIL. In addition, a more convincing demonstration that TIL, in at least some solid tumors, represents a better source effectors than PBL, is still lacking in humans, although it exists for experimental animal models.[8]

There might be advantages and potentially important therapeutic benefits to the use of TIL for immunotherapy. Exquisite specificity and effectiveness of immunologic reagents provide an attractive therapeutic goal. It has been suggested that AuTu-specificity of TIL might be their most attractive therapeutic attribute, especially if AuTu-specific CTL can be reliably generated in culture in numbers sufficient for therapy. Even if it were feasible to do so on the routine basis, therapy with TIL will not and probably should not be indiscriminately available to all patients with solid tumors. For example, patients might be considered eligible only if their tumors are: (a) well-infiltrated with TIL and (b) immunogenic on the basis of in vitro assays such as AuTu cytotoxicity.[53,54] Intensive efforts are being made to improve culture conditions for TIL and to selectively and consistently expand AuTu-specific effectors from TIL. These range from new cytokine combinations, e.g., IL-2, IL-4 and IL-7,[28,29,55,56] hollow fiber-based technology for growth of TIL,[12] attempts at improving antigen presentation in association with the relevant class I MHC antigen;[57] selection of $CD8^+$ or $CD4^+$ populations by panning prior to or after expansion of TIL in culture;[39,40] to gene transfer aimed at altering TIL growth characteristics in vitro.[58] Future improvements in therapy might focus on two separate approaches: one aimed at modification of the tumor to make it a better target for adoptively-transferred TIL and local immune cells, the other at improving clinical efficacy of TIL. A feasible approach in humans to modifying the tumor biology is delivery of cytokines to the tumor with the purpose of: (a) altering surface properties of tumor cells by e.g., increasing expression of class I MHC antigens[59,60] or adherence molecules;[61] (b) changing tumor growth by e.g., up- or down-regulating growth factor receptors or causing tumor cell differentiation;[62] (c) activation of inflammatory or immune cells already present at the tumor site;[63] (d) allowing an influx of inflammatory or immune cells by inducing a local cytokine cascade including chemotactic factors;[64] and (e) changing blood vessel permeability or inducing vascular stasis in the tumor.[47] Theoretically, it might be possible in the future to target cytokine genes linked to viral vectors for delivery to tumor cells endowing them with a capability to release a given cytokine and alter the microenvironment.[65] TIL might also be used as vectors to deliver cytokines to the tumor site.[13] Attempts at converting TIL into better effector cells in vivo depend on TIL ability to localize to the sites of tumor growth and/or metastasis. An attractive alternative, at least initially, might be to depend on local or regional delivery to the tumor of genetically-engineered TIL to be better able to evaluate their in vivo effectiveness. As vehicles for transfer of cytokines or other factors capable of altering tumor growth or biologic characteristics, TIL, and especially CTL, may indeed prove to be clinically very important in the future (Table 4).

The major limitations in the use of TIL for therapy of human cancer are several: (a) not all tumors are infiltrated with MNC, and TIL recovery is dependent on the tumor type, size, degree of necrosis and other tumor characteristics; (b) TIL obtained from tumors which produce immunosuppressive factors may be unable to proliferate in vitro; (c) TIL obtained from metastatic tumors may fail to expand in culture; (d) optimal in vitro conditions for activation and growth of TIL, including combinations of cytokines, are not known and may have to be tailored to individual TIL preparations; (e) growth of AuTu-specific TIL cannot be consistently achieved in most human tumors with the exception of melanoma; (f) numbers of TIL currently used for therapy are very large (10^{10}), although the

Table 4. Future goals for adoptive immunotherapy (AIT) of human cancer with TIL

1. Extend TIL therapy to tumors other than melanoma or renal cell carcinoma and establish its efficacy
2. Establish guidelines for optimal TIL delivery:
   - phenotype and AuTu specificity
   - optimal number
   - optimal culture conditions
   - concurrent delivery and optimal dose of cytokines
   - systemic vs locoregional delivery
   - in vitro correlates of clinical response
3. Reduce cost of AIT
4. Evaluate genetically-engineered TIL for localization to the tumor and clinical efficacy

optimal number of TIL for clinical efficacy in vivo is not known. In vitro expansion of TIL is both costly and time consuming; (g) delivery of TIL to the tumor bed or metastases via the systemic route of administration results in tumor localization of only a small fraction of TIL, as determined in studies with ^{111}In-labeled TIL in patients with melanoma; (h) mechanisms of TIL antitumor activity in vivo are not yet established and a lack of a unifying hypothesis for TIL therapy limits rational designs of clinical trials.

If TIL represent AuTu-specific T cells, as appears to be the case in at least some melanomas, the challenge of expanding and maintaining in culture of such CTL for therapy clearly represents a challenge. While it might be possible with time to overcome some of the limitations associated with in vitro culture of these effector cells, a concern remains that tumor-specific immunotherapy with CTL may not be an optimal approach, even in melanoma, which have been noted to be responsive to biologic therapies. Human tumors, including melanomas, are antigenically-heterogenous,[66,67] and this heterogeneity results in part, from the tumor's ability to modulate its surface antigens.[68] This, in turn, introduces the possibility that a fraction of tumor cells not expressing the relevant antigen may not be recognized and eliminated by adoptively transferred CTL. Evidence for a preferential usage of certain TcR V α and/or V β genes by TIL-T, as discussed earlier, indicates that TIL-derived CTL clones or lines might have specificities restricted to certain antigenic determinants. The presence of these antigenic determinants on all tumor cells is an a priori requirement for successful therapy based on tumor cell lysis by adoptively transferred CTL. The second concern, based on well-documented evidence from studies with animals bearing immunogenic tumors,[69] relates to the possibility that in addition to CTL, a tumor will activate the suppressor immune pathways, which might downregulate not only TIL at the tumor site but also adoptively-transferred CTL. The more immunogenic the tumor is, the more likely a possibility for activation of immunosuppressive circuits in addition to immunostimulatory ones. The third concern is about timing of therapy with CTL derived from the tumor bed. By the time human tumors come to surgery and TIL are available for in vitro expansion, it might be altogether too late for CTL activation, because of tumor-induced immunosuppression selectively directed at the $CD8^+$ T cells.[70] But even if CTL are obtained in culture, their in vivo effectiveness following adoptive transfer might be severely and perhaps selectively curtailed in the immunosuppressive tumor environment. Thus, adoptive immunotherapy with AuTu-specific effectors derived from TIL appears to present a number of difficulties above those that might exist with adoptive transfers of TIL in general.

SUMMARY

Overall, a rationale for adoptive immunotherapy with TIL in humans appears to be based on solid experimental evidence in animal models of tumor metastases.[8] Few clinical trials with TIL have been completed, however, and more clinical results are needed to determine antitumor efficacy of human TIL. Neither the antitumor mechanism of systemically-transferred TIL nor their clinical effectiveness in patients with metastatic disease other than melanoma have been confirmed. Rosenberg and his colleagues have demonstrated that it is feasible and safe to administer cultured TIL to patients with cancer.[4,5] The way has been prepared for further clinical protocols with human TIL. Processing and culture of TIL for AIT requires a clinical laboratory capable of handling large cell numbers (up to 10^{11} cells) and complying with good laboratory practice requirements. Quality control of cellular products is an essential part of AIT protocols, and it is necessary to assure sterility, safety and optimal characteristics of TIL transferred to patients. Further studies are needed, however, in order to: (a) evaluate the use of purified subsets or even cloned populations of TIL. Selection of appropriate subpopulations should lead to considerably greater efficiency of immunotherapy; (b) evaluate the role of TIL-derived $CD4^+$ T cell lines or clones in adoptive immunotherapy. Favorable clinical responses have been associated with transfer of in vitro-activated $CD4^+$ TIL;[33] (c) study lesions before and after therapy with TIL to characterize the cells which reached the tumor site after the transfer. The technique of in situ hybridization with probes for mRNAs of cytokines, perforin, other cellular products or products of genes inserted into TIL should allow a better definition of cellular characteristics of TIL and of their localization in respect to the vascular elements and tumor cells; (d) compare melanoma with other solid tumors to obtain insights into why melanomas appear to be more responsive to TIL/IL-2 therapy; (e) develop better methods to expand functionally-active effector cells from small initial numbers of TIL; (f) obtain more insights into mechanisms of increased selective localization of transferred TIL into tumor metastasis. It is likely that AIT with TIL will be made more effective in the future by devising ways to activate or augment antitumor effects of transferred cells and by applying novel strategies such as genetic modifications or tumor targeting involving bispecific antibodies.

References

1. Mazumder A, Eberlein TJ, Grimm EA, Wilson DJ, Keenan AM, Aamodt R, Rosenberg SA. Phase I study of adoptive immunotherapy of human cancer with lectin-activated autologous mononuclear cells. Cancer 1984; 53:896-905.
2. Rosenberg SA, Lotze MT, Muul LM, Leitman S, Chang AE, Ettinghausen SE, Matory YL, Skibber JM, Shiloni E, Vetto JT, Seipp CA, Simpson C, Reichert CM. Observations on the systemic administration of autologous lymphokine-activated killer cells and recombinant interleukin 2 to patients with metastatic cancer. N Engl J Med 1985; 313:1485-1492.
3. Rosenberg SA, Lotze MT, Muul LM, Chang AE, Avis FP, Leitman S, Lineban WM, Robertson CN, Lee RE, Rubin JT, Seipp CA, Simpson CG, White DE. A progress report on the treatment of 157 patients with advanced cancer using lymphokine-activated killer cells and interleukin 2 or high-dose interleukin 2 alone. N Engl J Med 1987; 316:889-897.
4. Topalian SL, Solomon D, Avis FP, Chang AE, Freerksen DL, Linehan WM, Lotze MT, Robertson CN, Seipp CA, Simon P, Simpson CG, Rosenberg SA. Immunotherapy of patients with advanced cancer using tumor-infiltrating lymphocytes and recombinant interleukin-2: A pilot study. J Clin Oncol 1988; 6:839-853.
5. Rosenberg SA, Packard BS, Aebersold PM, Solomon D, Topalian SL, Toy ST, Simon P, Lotze MT, Yang JC, Seipp CA, Simpson C, Carter C, Bock S, Schwartzentruber D, Wei JP, White DE. Use of tumor-infiltrating lymphocytes and interleukin-2 in the immunotherapy of patients with metastatic melanoma. A preliminary report. N Engl J Med 1988; 319:1676-1680.
6. Grimm EA, Mazumder A, Zhang HZ, Rosenberg SA. Lymphokine activated killer cell phenomenon: I. Lysis of natural killer

resistant fresh solid tumor cells by interleukin 2-activated autologous human peripheral blood lymphocytes. J Exp Med 1982; 155:1823-1841.

7. Grimm EA, Ramsey KM, Mazumder A, Wilson DJ, Djeu JY, Rosenberg SA. Lymphokine activated killer cell phenomenon: II. The precursor cells are serologically distinct from peripheral T lymphocytes, memory CTL and NK cells. J Exp Med 1983; 157:884-897.
8. Rosenberg SA, Spiess P, Lafreniere R. A new approach to adoptive immunotherapy of cancer with tumor-infiltrating lymphocytes. Science 1986; 233:1318-1321.
9. Sondel PM, Sosman JA, Hank JA, Kohler PC, Storer B. Tumor-infiltrating lymphocytes and interleukin-2 in melanomas. N Engl J Med 1989; 320:1418-1419.
10. Whiteside TL, Herberman RB. Isolation and culturing of lymphocytes for cellular adoptive immunotherapy. In: Rose NR, DeMacario EC, Fahey JL, Friedman H, Penn GM., eds.Manual of Clinical Laboratory Immunology. Washington,DC: Amer.Soc.Microbiol., 1992: 820-823.
11. Topalian SL, Muul LM, Solomon D, Rosenberg SA. Expansion of human tumor-infiltrating lymphocytes for use in immunotherapy trials. J Immunol Methods 1987; 102:127-141.
12. Knazek R, Wu YW, Aebersold PM, Rosenberg SA. Culture of human tumor-infiltrating lymphocytes in hollow fiber bioreactors. J Immunol Methods 1990; 127:29-37.
13. Rosenberg SA, Aebersold P, Cornetta K, Kasid A, Morgan RA, Moen R, Karson EM, Lotze MT, Yang JC, Topalian SL, Merino MJ, Culver K, Miller AD, Blaese RM, Anderson WF. Gene transfer into humans: Immunotherapy of patients with advanced melanoma, using tumor-infiltrating lymphocytes modified by retroviral gene transduction. N Engl J Med 1990; 323:570-578.
14. West WH, Tauer KW, Yannelli JR, Marshall GD, Orr DW, Thurman GB, Oldham RK. Constant-infusion recombinant interleukin-2 in adoptive immunotherapy of advanced cancer. N Engl J Med 1987; 316:898-905.
15. Squdrelli-Saraceno M, Rivoltini L, Cantu G, Ravagni F, Parmiani G, Molinari R. Local adoptive immunotherapy of advanced head and neck tumors with LAK cells and interleukin 2. Tumori 1991; 76:566-571.
16. Hercend T, Farace F, Baume D, Charpentier F, Droz JP, Triebel F, Escudier B. Immunotherapy with lymphokine-activated natural killer cells and recombinant interleukin 2: A feasibility trial in metastatic renal cell carcinoma. J Biol Resp Mod 1990; 9:546-555.
17. Lotze MT, Kawakami Y, Rosenberg SA. Immunotherapy protocols at the National Cancer Institute: Current status and future prospects. In: Lymphokine Receptor Interactions. 1989: 153-162.
18. Weiss GR, Margolin KA, Aronson FR, Sznol M, Atkins MB, Dutcher JP, Gaynor ER, Doldt DH, Doroshow JH, Bar MH, Hawkins MJ, Demchak PA, Gucalp R, Fisher RI. A randomized phase II trial of continuous infusion interleukin-2 or bolus injection interleukin-2 plus lymphokine-activated killer cells for advanced renal cell carcinoma. J Clin Oncol 1992; 10:275-281.
19. Lotze MT, Chang AE, Seipp CA, Simpson C, Vetto JT, Rosenberg SA. High-dose recombinant interleukin-2 in the treatment of patients with disseminated cancer: Responses, treatment-related morbidity, and histologic findings. JAMA 1986; 256:3117-3129.
20. Rosenberg SA, Lotze MT, Yang JC, Topalian SL, Chang AE, Schwartzentruber DJ, Aebersold P, Leitman S, Linehan WM, Seipp CA, White DE, Steinberg SM. Prospective randomized trial of high-dose interleukin-2 alone or in conjunction with lymphokine-activated killer cells for the treatment of patients with advanced cancer. JNCI 1993; 85:622-632.
21. Topalian SL, Solomon D, Rosenberg SA. Tumor-specific cytolysis by lymphocytes infiltrating human melanomas. J Immunol 1989; 142:3714-3724.
22. Hom SS, Topalian SL, Simonis T, Mancini M, Rosenberg SA. Common expression of melanoma tumor-associated antigens recognized by human tumor-infiltrating lymphocytes: Analysis by human lymphocyte antigen restriction. J Immunother 1991; 10:153-164.

23. Heo DS, Whiteside TL, Johnson JT, Chen K, Barnes EL, Herberman RB. Long-term interleukin 2-dependent growth and cytotoxic activity of tumor-infiltrating lymphocytes (TIL) from human squamous cell carcinomas of the head and neck. Cancer Res 1987; 47:6353-6362.
24. Parmiani G, Anichini A, Fossati G. Cellular immune response against autologous human malignant melanoma: are in vitro studies providing a framework for a more effective immunotherapy? JNCI 1990; 82:361-370.
25. Sosman JA, Kohler PC, Hank J, Moore KH, Bechhofer R, Storer B, Sondel PM. Repetitive weekly cycles of recombinant human interleukin 2: Responses of renal carcinoma with acceptable toxicity. JNCI 1988; 80:60-63.
26. Bergmann L, Weidmann E, Mitrou PS, Runne U, Keilholz U, Bartsch HH, Franks CR. Interleukin-2 in combination with interferon-α in disseminated malignant melanoma and advanced renal cell carcinoma. A phase I/II study. Onkologie 1990; 13:137-140.
27. Mule JJ, Yang J, Shu S, Rosenberg SA. The antitumor efficacy of lymphokine-activated killer cells and recombinant interleukin-2 in vivo: Direct correlation between reduction of established metastases and cytolytic activity of lymphokine-activated killer cells. J Immunol 1986; 136:3899-3909.
28. Kawakami Y, Rosenberg SA, Lotze MT. Interleukin 4 promotes the growth of tumor-infiltrating lymphocytes cytotoxic for human autologous melanoma. J Exp Med 1988; 168:2183-2191.
29. Stotter H, Custer MC, Bolton ES, Guedez L, Lotze MT. IL-7 induces human lymphokine-activated killer cell activity and is regulated by IL-4. J Immunol 1991; 146:150-155.
30. Kradin RL, Kurnick JT, Lazarus DS, Preffer FI, Dubinett SM, Pinto CE, Gifford J, Davidson E, Grove B, Callahan RJ, Strauss HW. Tumor-infiltrating lymphocytes and interleukin-2 in treatment of advanced cancer. Lancet 1989; 1:577-580.
31. Bukowski RM, Sharfman W, Murthy S, Rayman P, Tubbs R, Alexander J, Budd T, Sergie JS, Bauer L, Gibson V, Stanley J, Boyett J, Pontes E, Finke J. Clinical results and characterization of tumor-infiltrating lymphocytes with or without recombinant interleukin-2 in human metastatic renal cell carcinoma. Cancer Res 1991; 51:4199-4205.
32. Oldham RK, Dillman RO, Yannelli JR, Barth NM, Maleckar JR, Sferruzza A, Cohen RJ, Minor DR, Spitler L, Birch R, West WH. Continuous infusion interleukin-2 and tumor-derived activated cells as treatment of advanced solid tumors: A National Biotherapy Study Group Trial. Mol Biother 1991; 3:68-73.
33. Dillman RO, Oldham RK, Barth NM, Cohen RJ, Minor DR, Birch R, Yannelli JR, Maleckar JR, Sferruzza A, Arnold J, West WH. Continuous interleukin-2 and tumor-infiltrating lymphocytes as treatment of advanced melanoma. A National Bio-therapy Study Group Trial. Cancer 1991; 68:1-8.
34. Rivoltini L, Arienti F, Belli F, Gambacorti-Passerini C, Cascinelli N, Parmiani G. In vitro preferential lysis of autologous melanoma by tumor-infiltrating lymphoyctes (TIL). Association with clinical response after immunotherapy with TIL and IL-2. Abstract #1943. Proc AACR 1992; 33:326.
35. Rosenberg SA, Lotze MT, Yang JC, Aebersold PM, Linehan WM, Seipp CA, White DE. Experience with the use of high-dose interleukin 2 in the treatment of 652 cancer patients. Ann Surg 1989; 210:474-485.
36. Siegel JP, Puri RK. Interleukin 2 toxicity. J Clin Oncol 1991; 9:694-704.
37. Marincola FM, Balkissoon J, Schwartzentruber DJ, Hom SS, Concepcion R, Marcus SG, Yannelli J, Topalian SL, Parkinson DR, Rosenberg SA. Hemodynamic effects of the administration of tumor-infiltrating lymphocytes to cancer patients. J Immunother 1993; 13:282-288.
38. Shimizu Y, Iwatsuki S, Herberman RB, Whiteside TL. Effects of cytokines on in vitro growth of tumor-infiltrating lymphocytes obtained from human primary and metastatic liver tumors. Cancer Immunol Immunother 1991; 32:280-288.
39. Morecki S, Topalian SL, Myers WW, Okrongly D, Okarma TB, Rosenberg SA. Separation and growth of human CD4+ and CD8+ tumor-infiltrating lymphocytes and peripheral blood mononuclear cells by direct

positive panning on covalently attached monoclonal antibody-coated flasks. J Biol Resp Mod 1990; 9:463-474.

40. Letessier E, Heo DS, Okarma T, Johnson JT, Herberman RB, Whiteside TL. Enrichment in tumor-reactive CD8+ T lymphocytes by positive selection from the blood and lymph nodes of patients with head and neck cancer. Cancer Res 1991; 51:3891-3899.
41. Aebersold P, Hyatt C, Johnson S, Hines K, Korcak L, Sanders M, Lotze M, Topalian S, Yang J, Rosenberg SA. Lysis of autologous melanoma cells by tumor-infiltrating lymphocytes: Association with clinical response. JNCI 1991; 83:932-937.
42. Marincola FM, Venzon D, White D, Rubin JT, Lotze MT, Simonis TB, Balkissoon J, Rosenberg SA, Parkinson DR. HLA association with response and toxicity in melanoma patients treated with interleukin 2-based immunotherapy. Cancer Res 1992; 52:6561-6566.
43. Fisher B, Packard BS, Read EJ, Carrasquillo JA, Carter CS, Topalian SL, Yang JC, Yolles P, Larson SM, Rosenberg SA. Tumor localization of adoptively transferred indium-111 labeled tumor-infiltrating lymphocytes in patients with metastatic melanoma. J Clin Oncol 1989; 7:250-261.
44. Griffith KD, Read EJ, Carrasquillo JA, Carter CS, Yang JC, Fisher B, Aebersold P, Packard BS, Yu MY, Rosenberg SA. In vivo distribution of adoptively transferred indium-111-labeled tumor-infiltrating lymphocytes and peripheral blood lymphocytes in patients with metastatic melanoma. JNCI 1989; 81:1709-1717.
45. Mukherji B, Arnbjarnarson O, Spitznagle LA, Hoffman J, Ergin MT, Spencer RP. Biodistribution of IN-111 labeled tumor sensitized autologous lymphocytes in cancer patients. Prog Clin Biol Res 1987; 244:325-334.
46. Whiteside TL, Herberman RB. Extravasation of antitumor effector cells. Invasion & Metastasis 1992; 12:128-146.
47. Sasaki A, Melder RJ, Whiteside TL, Herberman RB, Jain RK. Preferential localization of human adherent lymphokine-activated killer (A-LAK) cells in tumor microcirculation: A novel mechanism for adoptive immunotherapy. JNCI 1991; 83:433-437.
48. Chang AE, Yoshizawa H, Sakai K, Cameron MJ, Sondak VK, Shu S. Clinical observations on adoptive immunotherapy with vaccine-primed T-lymphocytes secondarily sensitized to tumor in vitro. Cancer Res 1993; 53:1043-1050.
49. Alexander RB, Rosenberg SA. Long-term survival of adoptively transferred tumor-infiltrating lymphocytes in mice. J Immunol 1990; 145:1615-1620.
50. Alexander RB, Rosenberg SA. Adoptively transferred tumor-infiltrating lymphocytes can cure established metastatic tumor in mice and persist long-term in vivo as functional memory T lymphocytes. J Immunother 1991; 10:389-397.
51. Teare GF, Horan PK, Slezak SE, Smith C, Hay JB. Long-term tracking of lymphocytes in vivo: The migration of PKH-labeled lymphocytes. Cell Immunol 1991; 134:157-170.
52. Wallace PK, Palmer LD, Perry-Lalley D, Bolton ES, Alexander RB, Horan PK, Yang JC, Muirhead KA. Mechanisms of adoptive immunotherapy: Improved methods for in vivo tracking of tumor-infiltrating lymphoyctes and lymphokine-activated killer cells. Cancer Res 1993; 53:2358-2367.
53. Uchida A, Kariya Y, Okamoto N, Sugie K, Fujimoto T, Yagita M. Prediction of postoperative clinical course by autologous tumor-killing activity in lung cancer patients. Department of Late Effect Studies, Kyoto University, Japan. JNCI 1990; 82:1697-1701.
54. Ortaldo JR, Wiltrout RH. Implications of potential positive correlation between autologous tumor-cell-killing activity and prognosis in lung cancer. JNCI 1990; 82:1663-1665.
55. Lotze MT, Zeh HJ III, Elder EM, Cai Q, Pippin BA, Rosenstein MM, Whiteside TL, Herberman RB. Use of T-cell growth factors (interleukins 2, 4, 7, 10 and 12) in the evaluation of T-cell reactivity to melanoma. J Immunother 1992; 12:212-217.
56. Kawakami Y, Custer MC, Rosenberg SA, Lotze MT. IL-4 regulates IL-2 induction of lymphokine-activated killer activity from human lymphocytes. J Immunol 1989; 142:3452-3461.

57. Mortarini R, Belli F, Parmiani G, Anichini A. Cytokine-mediated modulation of HLA-class II, ICAM-1, LFA-3 and tumor-associated antigen profile of melanoma cells. Comparison with anti-proliferative activity by rIL-1-β, rTNF-α, rIFN-γ, rIL-4 and their combinations. Int J Cancer 1990; 45:334-341.
58. Kasid A, Morecki S, Aebersold P, Cornetta K, Culver K, Freeman S, Director E, Lotze MT, Blaese RM, Anderson WF, Rosenberg SA. Human gene transfer: Characterization of human tumor-infiltrating lymphocytes as vehicles for retroviral-mediated gene transfer in man. PNAS USA 1990; 87:473-477.
59. Vanky F, Stuber G, Rotstein S, Klein E. Autotumor recognition following in vitro induction of MHC antigen expression on solid human tumors: Stimulation of lymphocytes and generation of cytotoxicity against the original MHC-antigen-negative tumor cells. Cancer Immunol Immunother 1989; 28:17-21.
60. Taramelli D, Fossati G, Mazzocchi A, Delia D, Ferrone S, Parmiani G. Classes I and II HLA and melanoma-associated antigen expression and modulation on melanoma cells isolated from primary and metastatic lesions. Cancer Res 1986; 46:433-439.
61. Anichini A, Mortarini R, Supino R, Parmiani G. Human melanoma cells with high susceptibility to cell-mediated lysis can be identified on the basis of ICAM-1 phenotype, VLA profile and invasive ability. Int J Cancer 1990; 46:508-515.
62. Borden EC, Sondell PM. Lymphokines and cytokines in cancer treatment immunotherapy realized. Cancer 1990; 65:800-814.
63. Rosenberg SA. Immunotherapy of cancer using interleukin 2: Current status and future prospects. Immunol Today 1988; 9:58-62.
64. Van Damme J, Proost P, Lenaerts JP, Opdenakker G. Structural and functional identification of two human, tumor-derived monocyte chemotactic proteins (MCP-2 and MCP-3) belonging to the chemokine family. J Exp Med 1992; 176:59-65.
65. Russell SJ. Lymphokine gene therapy for cancer. Immunol Today 1990; 11:196-200.
66. Anichini A, Mazzocchi A, Fossati G, Parmiani G. Cytotoxic T lymphocyte clones from peripheral blood and from tumor site detect intratumor heterogeneity of melanoma cells. Analysis of specificity and mechanisms of interaction. J Immunol 1989; 142:3692-3701.
67. Houghton AN, Real FX, Davis LJ, Cordon-Cardo C, Old LJ. Phenotypic heterogeneity of melanoma. Relation to the differentiation program of melanoma cells. J Exp Med 1987; 165:812-829.
68. Johnson JP, Stade BG, Holzmann B, Schwable W, Riethmuller G. De novo expression of intercellular-adhesion molecule 1 in melanoma correlates with increased risk of metastasis. PNAS USA 1989; 86:641-644.
69. Bear HD. Tumor-specific suppressor T-cells which inhibit the in vitro generation of cytolytic T-cells from immune and early tumor-bearing host spleens. Cancer Res 1986; 46:1805-1812.
70. Miescher S, Stoeck M, Qiao L, Barras C, Barrelet L, Von Fliedner V. Preferential clonogenic deficit of CD8+ T lymphocytes infiltrating human solid tumors. Cancer Res 1988; 48:6992-6998.

INDEX

Items in italics denote figures (f) and tables (t).

A

Adhesion molecules, 19-20
Adoptive immunotherapy (AIT), 2, 89-90
  clinical trials, 98-100
  criteria, 103
  future, 103-105
  generation of autotumor-specific TIL, 100-101
  genetically modified TIL, 102-103
  localization to tumors, 101-102
  preparation of TIL, 90-94
  TIL/IL-2 vs IL-2 alone, 94, 96-98
Alexander JP, 43, 44, 53, 56, 57, 58
Anergy, 58, 83-84
Anichini A, 72
Antigen presentation, 59
Atopic dermatitis, 44
Autotumor (AuTu) -specific effector cells, 1. See Adoptive immunotherapy (AIT).

B

B lymphocytes, 11
Boon T, 73
Breast carcinoma, 10, 11
  c-erb B2 oncogene, 13
  estrogen receptors (ER), 12
  histopathology, *13t*
  immunohistology, 12-13
  in situ hybridization, 21, 23
  mucin-producing, 12-13, *14f-t*
Bretscher P, 83
Bukowski RM, 99

C

Cohen M, 83
Colon carcinoma
  immunohistology, 17-18
Cultured TIL, 67-68
  clonal analysis of, 72-73
  cytokine production by, 73-74
  expansion with combined cytokines, 69-70
    IL-2, 68-69
  outgrowth of AuTu-specific CTL from, 70-71
Cyclophosphamide, 99
Cytokines, 56
  expansion of cultured TIL with, 67-75
  genes, 10
    in situ hybridization for expression in TIL, 20-21, *22f*, 23-26, 56
  gene transfer into TIL, 3
  tumors and, 2, 11, 26
Cytotoxic T lymphocytes (CTL), 1, 74
  clonal analysis of, 72-73
  mucin-specific, 71
  outgrowth of AuTu-specific CTL from cultured TIL, 70-71, 100-101

D

Dillman RO, 48

E

Endothelial cell, 44-45
Epstein-Barr virus (EBV), 73

F

Feinberg AP, 21
Ferrarini M, 45
Ferrone S, 19
Fibronectin, 43
Finke JH, 61
Finn OJ, 71
Fisher B, 101
Functional characteristics of isolated TIL, 52
  activation by anti-CD3 or anti-CD28 monoclonal antibodies (mAbs), 57
  cytokine production, 56
  immunocompetence, 57-60
  limitations of functional studies, 52-53
  locomotion, 55-56
  proliferation and cytotoxicity, 53-55
  tumor interactions and, 60-61

G

Gallo RC, 11
Gene transfer, 94, *95f*

cytokine, 3
Granulocyte monocyte-colony stimulating factor (GM-CSF), 73, 100
Grave's disease, 44
Griffith KD, 101
Guerry D, 70

H

Hom SS, 73
House AK, 1

I

Immune suppression, 59, 60-61
tumor-associated antigens (TAA) as self-antigens, 84
In situ characterization of TIL
histopathology, 7, 10-11
immunohistology, 8-10, 11-12
breast carcinoma, 12-13
colon carcinoma, 17-18
liver tumors
primary, 18-20
melanoma, 12
ovarian carcinoma, 15, *16f*, 17
squamous cell carcinoma of the head and neck (SCCHN), 13-15
in situ hybridization (ISH), 10
cytokine gene expression, 20-21, *22f*, 23-26
Integrin, 43
Interferon (IFN)
-a, 103
-g, 23, 24, 26, 56, 59, 69, 70, 73, 74, 100
Interleukin
-1, 24, 56, 70
-2, 2, 21, 26, 43, 56, 57, 58, 59, 60, 61, 67, 73, 83
adoptive immunotherapy (AIT) and, 89-90, 94, 96-100
expansion of cultures TIL with, 68-69
up-regulation of antitumor responses, 84-85
-4, 26, 69, 70, 73, 98
-6, 73
-7, 69, 98
Ioachim HL, 1
Isolation of TIL, 32
banking of TIL and tumor cells, 33-34
evaluation of purity and recovery, 35-37
gradients for separation of TIL and tumor cells, 34-35
tissue collection and processing, 32-33

J

Jerne NK, 26

K

Kaposi's sarcoma, 11
Klein E, 34
Koo AS, 74

L

Leishmania braziliensis, 44
Leprosy, 44
Lewis CE, 26
Liver tumors
primary
CD4/CD8 ratio, *43t*
immunohistology, 18-20
TcR, 46-47
Lotze MT, 94, 98
Lung cancer, 19
g/d TcR, 45
Lymphoid suppressor cells, 59
Lymphokine-activated killer (LAK) cell, 2, 3, 74, 89-90, 94, 96, 97

M

MacCarty WC, 1
Macrophages
tumor-associated (TAM), 39
Major histocompatibility complex (MHC), 19
cytotoxic T lymphocytes and, 71, 100-101
restriction, 82
Marincola FM, 100
Melanoma, 2, 10, *12f*, *34t*, 44, 70, 71, 73
adoptive immunotherapy (AIT), 89-90, 96
clinical trials, 98-100
genetically modified TIL, 102-103
immunohistology, 12
major histocompatibility complex (MHC), 19
TcR and, 46, 47-48
tumor-associated antigen, 83
Memory T cells, 43-45
Metastases
adoptive immunotherapy (AIT), 99
expansion of cultures TIL from, 68, *69f*
functional characteristics of isolated TIL, 55, 58, 60-61
Miescher S, 53
Mononuclear cells (MNC). See also Tumor-infiltrating lymphocytes.
infiltrates in tumors, 1, 2, 10-11
Morphologic and phenotypic characteristics of isolated TIL, 39
morphology, 39-40
phenotypic analysis
two-color flow cytometry, 40-41
Mukherji B, 59, 71, 101

Mule J, 98
Multiple sclerosis, 44

N

Natural killer (NK) cells, 11, 26, 45, 61, 74
Neomycin resistance gene (NeoR), 3, 94, 102-103

O

Ovarian carcinoma, 10, 45, 58
  immunohistology, 15, *16f,* 17
  in situ hybridization, 23

P

Parmiani G, 72
Peripheral blood lymphocytes (PBL), 53, 103
Phenotypic characteristics of isolated TIL. See
  Morphologic and phenotypic characteristics
    of isolated TIL.
Poggi A, 19
Polymerase chain reaction (PCR), 25-26
Polymorphic epithelial mucins (PEM), 82
Pretlow TG, 34
Pretlow TP, 34
Prostaglandin E_2 (PGE_2), 70
Pupa SM, 11

R

Renal cell carcinoma (RCC), 2, 11, 19, 73
  adoptive immunotherapy (AIT), 90, 96
    clinical trials, 98-100
Retrovirus, 94, 102-103
Reverse hemolytic plaque assay (RHPA), 26
Rheumatoid arthritis, 44
Rosen PP, 11
Rosenberg SA, 2, 89, 96, 97, 100, 101, 102, 106
Rubin JT, 84

S

Schoof DJ, 57
Schwartz RH, 83
Signal transduction, 61
Squamous cell carcinoma of the head and neck
  (SCCHN), 10, 61
  CD4/CD8 ratio, 41, *42t*
  cytokine production, *56t*
  immunohistology, 13-15
  in situ hybridization, *23f,* 24
Svennevig JL, 1

T

T cell receptor (TcR), 20, 27, *45f*
  g/d, 45
  gene usage by TIL in situ, 45-48
Thyroid carcinoma, 11
T lymphocytes, 27
  activated in TIL, 43
  CD3, 41, 57, 61
  CD3CD8, 69-70, 100
  CD4/CD8 ratio, 11, 15, 41-43
    cytokine production, 73
  CD25, 11, 41
  CD28, 57
  CD29, 43-45
  CD45, 43-45
  memory, 43-45
  tumor surveillance, 81-82
    recognition of tumor-associated antigens (TAA) by T cells, 82-84
    tumor-associated antigens (TAA) as self-antigens, 84
    tumor-specific T cells, 82
    up-regulation of antitumor responses, 84-85
Transferrin receptor (CD71), 43
Transforming growth factor (TGF) b, 70
Tuberculous granulomas, 44
Tumor-associated antigen (TAA), 2, 27, 71, 81
Tumor necrosis factor
  a (TNF-a), 21, 24, 56, 60, 69, 70, 73, 74, 94, 100, 103
  b (TNF-b), 21, 23, *25f,* 60, 73
Tyrosine kinases, 61

U

Uchida A, 103
Underwood JCE, 1

V

Vogelstein B, 21
Vose BM, 34

W

Wallace PK, 102
Watt AG, 1
Weidmann E, 47

Z

Zocchi MR, 19, 45, 57